MEDICAL TERMINOLOGY CHEAT SHEET

The Big Book of Medical Terminology Workbook

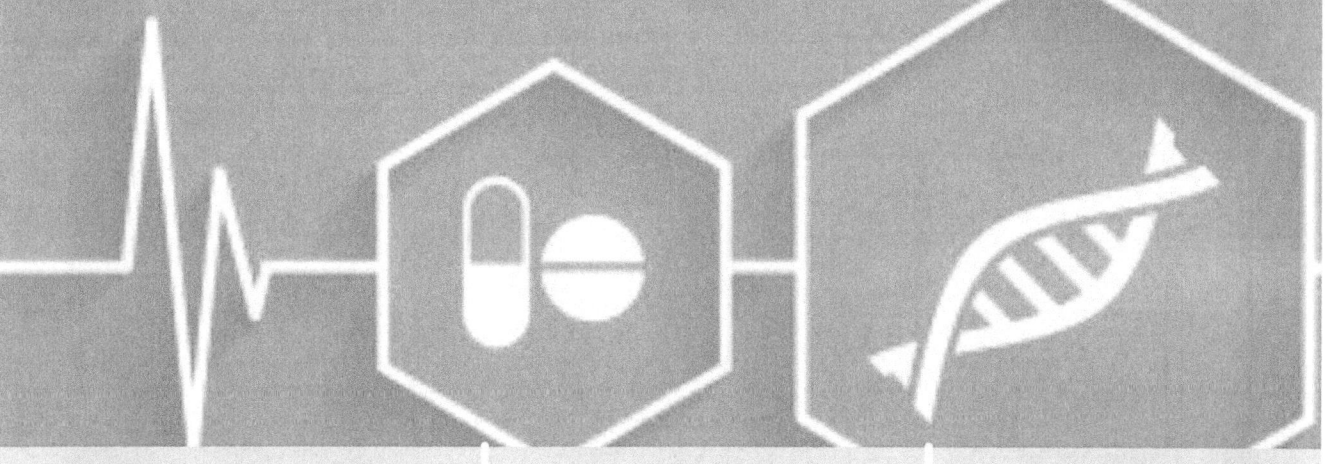

2900+ Terms	Prefixes	Suffixes
Root Words	Abbreviations	Word Search
Crosswords	Quiz	Test

APPENDIX A: Medical Terminology

National EMS Education Standard Competencies

Medical Terminology

Uses foundational anatomical and medical terms and abbreviations in written and oral communication with colleagues and other health care professionals.

Medical Terminology

It is critical that you have a strong working knowledge of medical terminology. The language of medicine is primarily derived from Greek and Latin. Medical terminology is used in international language, and it is also necessary for communicating with other medical personnel. The wider your vocabulary base, the more competent you seem to the rest of the medical community and the better the patient care you will be able to provide. Understanding terminology involves breaking words down into their separate components of prefix, suffix, and root word and having a good working knowledge of those parts.

Prefixes

A prefix appears at the beginning of a word and generally describes location and intensity. Prefixes are frequently found in general language (ie, autopilot, submarine, tricycle), as well as in medical and scientific terminology. When a medical word (ventilation) contains a prefix (hyper), the meaning of the word is altered (hyperventilation). Not all medical terms have prefixes.

By learning to recognize a few of the more commonly used medical prefixes, you can figure out the meanings of terms that may not be immediately familiar to you. **Table A-1** lists common prefixes.

Suffixes

Suffixes are placed at the end of words to change the original meaning. In medical terminology, a suffix usually indicates a procedure, condition, disease, or part of speech.

A commonly used suffix is -itis, which means "inflammation." When this suffix is paired with the prefix arthro-, meaning joint, the resulting word is arthritis, an inflammation of the joints. Sometimes it is necessary to change the last letter or letters of the root word or prefix when a suffix is added to make pronunciation easier. **Table A-2** lists common suffixes.

Root Words

The main part or stem of a word is called a root word. A root word conveys the essential meaning of the word and frequently indicates a body part. With a combining form, the root word and a combining vowel such as i, e, o, or a may be combined with another root word, a prefix, or a suffix to describe a particular structure or condition.

A frequently used term in EMS is CPR, which stands for cardiopulmonary resuscitation. When we break it down, cardio is a root word meaning "heart," and pulmonary is a root word meaning "lungs." By performing CPR we introduce air into the lungs and circulate blood by compressing the heart to resuscitate the patient. Some root words may also be used as prefixes or suffixes; those already appear in the earlier tables. **Table A-3** lists common root words.

Abbreviations

Abbreviations take the place of words to shorten notes or documentation. When you are using abbreviations in patient care reports, remember to use only standard, accepted abbreviations to avoid confusion and errors. **Table A-4** lists commonly used abbreviations. This list is intended to help you decipher documents written by other health care professionals. Before using any abbreviations in your own reports, you should be familiar with accepted use of abbreviations in your local jurisdiction or service area.

Table A-1 Common Prefixes

Prefix	Meaning	Prefix	Meaning	Prefix	Meaning
a-	without, lack of	cyst(o)-	pertaining to the bladder or any fluid-containing sac	inter-	between
ab-	away from	cyt(o)-	pertaining to a cell	intra-	within
abdomi(n)-	abdomen	de-	down from	iso-	equal
acr(o)-	pertaining to an extremity	dermat(o)-	pertaining to the skin	latero-	side
ad-	to, toward	di-	twice, double	leuk(o)-	pertaining to anything white or to leukocytes (white blood cells)
aden(o)-	pertaining to a gland	dia-	through, completely	lith(o)-	pertaining to a stone
an-	without, lack of	dys-	difficult, painful, abnormal	macro-	large
ana-	up, back, again	ect(o)-	out from	mal-	bad or abnormal
angio-	vessel	electro-	pertaining to electricity	medi-	middle
ante-	before, forward	end(o)-	within	mega-	large
anti-	against, opposed to	enter(o)-	pertaining to the intestines	melan-	black
arteri(o)-	artery	epi-	upon, on	mening(o)-	pertaining to a membrane, particularly the meninges
arthro-	pertaining to a joint	erythr(o)-	pertaining to anything red or to erythrocytes (red blood cells)	micro-	small
auto-	self	eu-	easy, good, normal	mono-	one
bi-	two	ex(o)-	outside	myel(o)-	pertaining to the spinal cord, the bone marrow, or myelin
bi(o)-	pertaining to life	extra-	outside, in addition	my(o)-	pertaining to muscle
blast(o)-	germ or cell	gastr(o)-	pertaining to the stomach	nas(o)-	pertaining to the nose
blephar(o)-	pertaining to an eyelid	glyc(o)-	sugar	ne(o)-	new
brady-	slow	gynec(o)-	pertaining to females or the female reproductive organs	nephr(o)-	pertaining to the kidney
calc-	stone; also heel	hemat(o)-	pertaining to blood	neur(o)-	pertaining to a nerve or the nervous system
cardi(o)-	pertaining to the heart	hemi-	half	noct-	night
cephal(o)-	pertaining to the head	hem(o)-	pertaining to blood	olig(o)-	little, deficient
cerebr(o)-	pertaining to the cerebrum, a part of the brain	hepat(o)-	pertaining to the liver	oophor(o)-	pertaining to the ovary
cervic(o)-	pertaining to the neck or the uterine cervix	heter-	other, different	ophthalm(o)-	pertaining to the eye
chole-	pertaining to bile	hom-	same or like	orchid(o)-	pertaining to the testicles
chondr(o)-	pertaining to cartilage	hydr(o)-	water	orchi(o)-	pertaining to the testicles
circum-	around, about	hyper-	over, excessive	oro-	pertaining to the mouth
contra-	against, opposite	hypo-	under, deficient	ortho-	straight or normal
cost(o)-	pertaining to a rib	hyster(o)-	pertaining to the uterus	oste(o)-	pertaining to bone
cyan(o)-	blue	infra-	below	ot(o)-	pertaining to the ear

▼ *continues*

Appendix A Medical Terminology

Table A-1 Common Prefixes, continued

Prefix	Meaning	Prefix	Meaning	Prefix	Meaning
para-	by the side of	pseud(o)-	false	semi-	half or partial
path(o)-	pertaining to disease	psych(o)-	pertaining to the mind	sub-	under, moderately
per-	through	pulm(o)-	pertaining to the lung	super-	above, excessive, or more than normal
peri-	around	pur-	pertaining to pus	supra-	above
phag(o)-	pertaining to eating, ingesting, or engulfing	pyel(o)-	pertaining to the kidney or pelvis	tachy-	fast
pharyng(o)-	pertaining to the throat, or pharynx	py(o)-	pertaining to pus	therm-	pertaining to temperature
phleb(o)-	pertaining to a vein	quadr(i)-	four	thorac(o)-	pertaining to the chest
pneum(o)-	pertaining to respiration, the lungs, or air	quar-	four	trans-	across
poly-	many	quat-	four	tri-	three
post-	after, behind	retr(o)-	backward or behind	uni-	one
pre-	before	rhin(o)-	pertaining to the nose	vas(o)-	vessel
pro-	before, in front of	salping(o)-	pertaining to a tube		
proct(o)-	pertaining to the rectum	scler(o)-	hard; also means pertaining to the sclera		

Table A-2 Common Suffixes

Suffix	Meaning	Suffix	Meaning	Suffix	Meaning
-algia	pertaining to pain	-emia	pertaining to the presence of a substance in the blood	-ology	science of
-asthen(o)	weakness	-genic	causing	-oma	tumor
-blast	immature cell	-gram	record	-osis	pertaining to a disease process (see also -sis)
-cele	pertaining to a tumor or swelling	-graph	a record or the instrument used to create the record	-ostomy	surgical creation of an opening, or hole
-centesis	pertaining to a procedure in which an organ or body cavity is punctured, often to drain excess fluid or obtain a sample for analysis	-itis	inflammation	-otomy	surgical incision
-cyte	cell	-lysis	decline, disintegration, or destruction	-pathy	disease or a system for treating disease
-ectomy	surgical removal of	-megaly	enlargement of	-phagia	pertaining to eating or swallowing

▼ continues

Table A-2 Common Suffixes, continued

Suffix	Meaning	Suffix	Meaning	Suffix	Meaning
-phasia	pertaining to speech	-rrhage	abnormal or excessive flow or discharge	-sis	a process, action, or condition
-phobia	pertaining to an irrational fear	-rrhagia	abnormal or excessive flow or discharge	-taxis	order, arrangement of
-plasty	plastic surgery	-rrhaphy	suture of; repair of	-trophic	pertaining to nutrition
-plegia	paralysis	-rrhea	flow or discharge	-uria	pertaining to a substance in the urine or the condition so indicated
-pnea	pertaining to breathing	-scope	instrument for examination		
-ptosis	drooping	-scopy	examination with an instrument		

Table A-3 Common Root Words

Root Word	Meaning	Root Word	Meaning	Root Word	Meaning
acou-	hear	carotid	great arteries of the neck	gest-	carry, produce, congestion
adip-	fat	carpus	wrist	gno-	know
alb-	white	cent-	a fraction in the metric system; one hundredth or 100	-gram	something written or recorded
alges-	pain	cente-	to puncture (a body cavity)	graph-	write, record
andr-	male	cili-	eyelid	humerus	the bone in the upper arm
aorta	large artery exiting from the left ventricle of the heart	cleid(o)-	clavicle	idi-	separate, distinct
aqua-	water	cubitus	elbow	iod(o)-	iodine
asphyxia	lack of oxygen or excess of carbon dioxide in the body that results in unconsciousness	cycl-	circle or cycle	lact-	milk
asthen-	weak	digit	finger or toe	lingu-	tongue
audi-	to hear	ede-	swelling	men-	month
bronch-	windpipe	-esthesi(o)-	pertaining to sensation or perception	ocul-	eye
bucc-	cheek	febr-	fever	ov-	egg
bursa	pouch or sac	flex	bend	palpate	to examine by touch
callus	hard, thick skin; also a meshwork of connective tissue that forms during the healing process after a fracture	foramen	opening	ped-	child or foot
carcin-	cancer	fract-	break	percuss	to examine by striking

▼ continues

Table A-3 Common Root Words, continued

Root Word	Meaning	Root Word	Meaning	Root Word	Meaning
phot-	light	sepsis	the presence of microorganisms or their toxins in the blood; also the toxic condition caused by such presence	tom-	cut
pleur-	rib, side	sept-	wall, divider; also seven	toxic	poisonous
pod-	foot	serum	the clear portion of body fluids, including blood	trich-	hair
pto-	fall	sinus	cavity, channel, or hollow space	ur-	urine
ptyal-	saliva	som(a)-	body	varic-	varicose vein
pyr-	fire	spir-	coil	vertigo	a disordered sensation in which one's own body or the surroundings are perceived as moving
radius	the forearm bone on the thumb side; also a line from the center of a circle or sphere to the edge	stasis	slowing or stopping of the normal flow of a fluid, such as blood	viscer-	internal organs
ren-	kidney	stature	height	viscous	sticky
retina	inner nerve-containing layer of the eye	stern(o)-	sternum (breastbone)	xen-	foreign (material)
sangui(n)-	blood	stoma	any small opening on the surface of the body, such as a pore; also, the opening created in the abdominal wall for the passage of urine or feces	xer-	dry
sebum	a fatty secretion of the sebaceous glands	tact-	touch		
sect-	cut	tetra-	four		

Table A-4 Common Abbreviations*

*Sometimes abbreviations are written with periods (for example, abd. and a.c.), and sometimes different capitalization might be used and might convey a different meaning. Not all possible meanings for the abbreviations in this table are given here. Unless you are certain about the meaning, ask the person who used the abbreviation.

Abbreviation	Meaning	Abbreviation	Meaning	Abbreviation	Meaning
A&P	anatomy and physiology	ACLS	advanced cardiac life support	AK	above the knee
ā	before	ad lib	as much as desired	AKA	above the knee amputation
āā	of each (used in writing prescriptions)	ADL	activity of daily living	A-line	arterial line
abd	abdomen	AED	automated external defibrillator	AMA	against medical advice
ABG	arterial blood gas	AF	atrial fibrillation	amb	ambulatory
ac	before meals	AIDS	acquired immunodeficiency syndrome	AMI	acute myocardial infarction

▼ continues

Table A-4 Common Abbreviations, continued

Abbreviation	Meaning	Abbreviation	Meaning	Abbreviation	Meaning
AMS	altered mental status	CABG	coronary artery bypass graft	CVP	central venous pressure
ant	anterior	CAD	coronary artery disease	CXR	chest x-ray
AO × 4	alert and oriented to person, place, time, and self	CBC	complete blood count	D&C	dilation and curettage
AP	anteroposterior, front-to-back, action potential, angina pectoris, anterior pituitary, arterial pressure	cc	cubic centimeter	D/C	discontinue
APC	atrial premature complex, activated protein C, aspirin-phenacetin-caffeine	CC or C/C	chief complaint	diff	differential
Aq	water	CCU	coronary care unit	dig	digoxin
ARDS	adult respiratory distress syndrome	CHF	congestive heart failure	DM	diabetes mellitus
ASA	aspirin (acetylsalicylic acid)	Cl^-	chloride	DOA	dead on arrival
ASAP	as soon as possible	cm	centimeter	DOE	dyspnea on exertion
ASHD	arteriosclerotic or atherosclerotic heart disease	cm^3	cubic centimeter	DON	director of nursing
AV, A-V	atrioventricular, arteriovenous	CNS	central nervous system	DOS	dead on scene
BBB	bundle branch block	c/o	complaining of	DPT	diphtheria, pertussis, and tetanus toxoids vaccine
bid	twice daily	CO	cardiac output, carbon monoxide	DSD	dry sterile dressing
BKA	below the knee amputation	CO_2	carbon dioxide	DtaP	diphtheria, tetanus toxoids, and acellular pertussis vaccine
BM	bowel movement	COLD	chronic obstructive lung disease	DTP	diphtheria, tetanus toxoids, and pertussis vaccine
BP	blood pressure	COPD	chronic obstructive pulmonary disease	DTs	delirium tremens
BS	blood sugar, breath sounds, bowel sounds, bachelor of science (degree)	CP	chest pain, chemically pure, cerebral palsy	DVT	deep venous thrombosis
BSA	body surface area	CPR	cardiopulmonary resuscitation	D_5W	dextrose 5% in water
bx	biopsy	CRNA	certified registered nurse anesthetist	Dx	diagnosis
$\bar{c}$	with	CRT	capillary refill time, cathode-ray tube	ECG	electrocardiogram
°C	degrees Celsius (centigrade)	CSF	cerebrospinal fluid	ED	emergency department
Ca	calcium	CSM	carotid sinus massage, cerebrospinal meningitis	EDC	estimated date of confinement
CA	cancer, cardiac arrest, chronologic age, coronary artery, cold agglutinin	CVA	cerebrovascular accident	EEG	electroencephalogram

▼ continues

Table A-4 Common Abbreviations, continued

Abbreviation	Meaning	Abbreviation	Meaning	Abbreviation	Meaning
eg	for example	h	hour	JVD	jugular venous distention
EKG	electrocardiogram	(H)	hypodermic	K^+	potassium
ENT	ears, nose, and throat	H	hypodermic	KCl	potassium chloride
ER	emergency room	H&H	hemoglobin and hematocrit	kg	kilogram
ET	endotracheal tube, endotracheal	H&P	history and physical	KUB	kidneys, ureters, and bladder
ETA	estimated time of arrival	H/A	headache	KVO	keep vein open
ETOH	ethyl alcohol	Hb	hemoglobin	L	liter
ETT	endotracheal tube	Hct	hematocrit	LAC	laceration, laparoscopic-assisted colectomy
°F	degrees Fahrenheit	Hg	mercury	lb	pound
F_{IO_2}	fraction of inspired oxygen	Hgb	hemoglobin	LE	lower extremity, left eye, lupus erythematosus
FBS	fasting blood sugar	HH	hiatal hernia	LLL	left lower lobe of the lung
Fe	iron	HIV	human immunodeficiency virus	LLQ	left lower quadrant of the abdomen
FHR	fetal heart rate	H_2O	water	L/M	liters per minute
FHT	fetal heart tones	H_2O_2	hydrogen peroxide	LMP	last menstrual period
FHx	family history	HPI	history of present illness	LOC	level of consciousness, loss of consciousness
fL	femtoliter	hr	hour	LPM	liters per minute
fl	fluid	hs	at bedtime	LPN	licensed practical nurse
fld	fluid	HTN	hypertension	LR	lactated Ringer's
FSH	follicle-stimulating hormone	Hx	history	LSD	lysergic acid diethylamide
fx	fracture	Hz	hertz	LUL	left upper lobe of the lung
g	gram	I&O	intake and output	LUQ	left upper quadrant of the abdomen
GB	gallbladder	IC	intracardiac, inspiratory capacity, irritable colon	LVN	licensed vocational nurse
GI	gastrointestinal	ICP	intracranial pressure	m	meter
gm	gram	ICU	intensive care unit	MAE	moves all extremities
gr	grain	IDDM	insulin-dependent diabetes mellitus	MAEW	moves all extremities well
GSW	gunshot wound	IM	intramuscular	MAP	mean arterial pressure
gtt	drop(s)	IO	intraosseous	mcg	microgram
GTT	glucose tolerance test	IPPB	intermittent positive pressure breathing	MCL	midclavicular line, modified chest lead
GU	genitourinary	IUD	intrauterine (contraceptive) device	mEq	milliequivalent
gyn	gynecology	IV	intravenous	mg	milligram (mgm is a former symbol)

▼ *continues*

Table A-4 Common Abbreviations, continued

Abbreviation	Meaning	Abbreviation	Meaning	Abbreviation	Meaning
MI	myocardial infarction	NKDA	no known drug allergies	PE	pulmonary embolism, physical examination
MICU	mobile intensive care unit; medical intensive care unit	NPA	nasopharyngeal airway	PEA	pulseless electrical activity
min	minute	NPO	nil per os (nothing by mouth)	PEARL	pupils equal and reactive to light
mL	milliliter	NS	normal saline	ped(s)	pediatric
mm	millimeter	NSR	normal sinus rhythm	PEEP	positive end-expiratory pressure
mm Hg	millimeters of mercury	NTG	nitroglycerin	PERL	pupils equal and reactive to light
MRI	magnetic resonance imaging	N/V	nausea and vomiting	PERRL	pupils equal, round, and reactive to light
MS	morphine sulfate, multiple sclerosis	N/V/D	nausea, vomiting, and diarrhea	pH	hydrogen ion concentration
MSO_4	morphine sulfate	NVD	neck vein distention	PID	pelvic inflammatory disease
MVA	motor vehicle accident	O_2	oxygen	PND	paroxysmal nocturnal dyspnea
MVC	motor vehicle crash	OB	obstetrics	po	per os (by mouth)
MVP	mitral valve prolapse	OBS	organic brain syndrome	PO	postoperative, "post op"
N	normal	OD	overdose, right eye, optical density, outside diameter, doctor of optometry	Po_2	partial pressure of oxygen
Na	sodium	OP	outpatient	PRN	pro re nata (as needed)
NA, N/A	not applicable	OPA	oropharyngeal airway	psi	pounds per square inch
NaCl	sodium chloride	OR	operating room	PSVT	paroxysmal supraventricular tachycardia
NAD	no apparent distress, no appreciable disease	OS	left eye	pt	patient
$NaHco_3$	sodium bicarbonate	OU	both eyes	PT	physical therapy
NC	nasal cannula	oz	ounce	PTA	prior to admission, plasma thromboplastin antecedent
NG	nasogastric	$\bar{p}$	after	PTT	partial thromboplastin time
NICU	neonatal intensive care unit	pc	after meals	PVC	premature ventricular complex, polyvinyl chloride
NIDDM	non-insulin-dependent diabetes mellitus	Pco_2	partial pressure of carbon dioxide	PVD	peripheral vascular disease
NKA	no known allergies	PDR	*Physicians' Desk Reference*	q	every

▼ continues

Table A-4 Common Abbreviations, continued

Abbreviation	Meaning	Abbreviation	Meaning	Abbreviation	Meaning
qd	every day	stat	immediately	WBC	white blood cell
qh	every hour	STD	sexually transmitted disease	WNL	within normal limits
qid	four times a day	Sub Q	subcutaneous	w/o	without
qod	every other day	SVT	supraventricular tachycardia	wt	weight
RA	rheumatoid arthritis, right atrium	Sx	symptoms	yo	year old
RAD	reactive airway disease, right axis deviation	sym	symptoms	$\bar{x}$	except
RBC	red blood cell	tab	tablet	1°	first, first degree, primary
Rh	Rhesus blood factor, rhodium	TB	tuberculosis	2°	secondary, second degree
RHD	rheumatic heart disease	TBA	to be admitted, to be announced	↑	increase(d)
RL	Ringer's lactate	tbsp	tablespoon	↓	decrease(d)
RLL	right lower lobe of the lung	tech	technician, technologist	∅	no, not, none
RLQ	right lower quadrant of the abdomen	TIA	transient ischemic attack	®	right
RN	registered nurse	tid	three times a day	Ⓒ	left
R/O	rule out	TKO	to keep open	μ	micro
ROM	range of motion, rupture of membranes	TPR	temperature, pulse, respiration	α	alpha
RUL	right upper lobe of the lung	tsp	teaspoon	β	beta
RUQ	right upper quadrant of the abdomen	Tx	treatment	~	approximately
Rx	prescription	U	unit	×2	times two
$\bar{s}$	without	UA	urinalysis	/	per
SC	subcutaneous, secretory component	UE	upper extremity	≠	not equal
SICU	surgical intensive care unit	URI	upper respiratory infection	>	greater than
SIDS	sudden infant death syndrome	USP	United States Pharmacopeia	<	less than
SL	sublingual	UTI	urinary tract infection	?	questionable, possible
SOB	shortness of breath	VD	venereal disease	Δ	change
SQ	subcutaneous	vol	volume	−	negative
ss	half	VS	vital signs	♀	female
S/S	signs and symptoms	w/	with	♂	male

Medical Terminology

Question Combining Forms	Answer
abdominal cavity	Body pace between abdominal walls, above the pelvis, and below the diaphragm.
abdomin(o)	abdomen
acetabul(o)	cut-shaped hip socket
aden(o)	gland
adip(o)	fat
adren(o)	adrenal glands
alveol(o)	air sac, alveolus
angi(o)	vessel
anterior	At or toward the front(of the body).
aort(o)	aorta
appendic(o)	appendix
arteri(o)	artery
arteriol(o)	arteriole a tiny artery connecting to a capillary.
arthr(o)	joint; articulation
aur(i), auricul(o)	ear
blephar(o)	eyelid
brachi(o)	arm
blood system	Body system that includes blood and all its component parts
bronch(o), bronchi	bronchus
bucc(o)	cheek
burs(o)_	bursa
calcane(o)	heel bone
cardi(o)	heart;esophageal opening of the stomach
cardiovascular system	Body system that includes the heart and blood vessels; circulatory system.
carp(o)	wrist bones
celi(o)	abdomen
cell	Smallest unit of a living structure
cephal(o)	head
cerebell(o)	cerebellum
cerebr(o)	cerebellum
cervic(o)	neck;cervix
cheil(o), chil(o)	lip
chir(o)	hand
chol(e), cholo	bile
chondri(o), chondro	cartilage
col(o), colon(o)	colon
colp(o)	vagina
connective tissue	Fibrous substance that forms the body's supportive framework.
core(o)	pupil

cranial cavity	Space in the head that contains the brain
cortic(o)	cortex
costi, costo	rib
crani(o)	cranium
cross-sectional plane	Imaginary line that insects the body horizontally.
cyst(i), cysto	bladder; cyst
cyt(o)	cell
dactyl(o)	fingers, toes
deep	Away from the surface (of the body).
dent(i), dento	tooth
derm(o), derma, dermat(o)	skin
diaphragm	Muscle that divides the abdominal and thoracic cavities.
digestive system	Body system that includes all organs of digestion and waste excretions, from the mouth to the anus.
distal	Away from the point of attachment of the trunk.
dorsal	At or toward the back of the body
dorsal cavity	Main cavity on the back side of the body containing the cranial and spinal cavities.
duoden(o)	duodenum
encephal(o)	brain
endocrine system	Body system that includes glands that secrete hormones to regulate certain body functions.
enter(o)	intestines
epigastic region	Area of the body immediately above the stomach.
episi(o)	vulva
epithelial tissue	Tissue that covers or lines the body or its parts.
frontal plane	Imaginary line that divides that body into anterior and posterior positions.
gastr(o)	stomach
gingiv(o)	gum
gloss(o)	tongue
gnath(o)	jaw
gonad(o)	sex glands
hem(a), hemat(o), hemo	blood
hemic system	Organs involved in the production of blood including the cellular and the molecular components essential in providing defenses against foreign organisms or substances.
hepat(o), hepatic(o)	liver
hidr(o)	sweat
histi(o), histo	tissue
hypochondriac regions	Left and right regions of the body just below the cartilage of the ribs and immediately above the abdomen.
hypogastric regions	Areas of the body just below the umbilical region.
hyster(o)	uterus, hysteria
ile(o)	ileum
ili(o)	ilium
iliac regions	Left and right regions of the body near the upper portions of the hip bone.
inferior	Below another body structure.

inguin(o)	groin
inguinal regions	Left and right regions of the body near the upper portion of the hip bone.
integumentary system	Body system that includes skin, hair, and nails.
irid(o)	iris
ischi(o)	ischium
kary(o)	nucleus
kerat(o)	cornea
labi(o)	lip
lamin(o)	lamina
lapar(o)	abdominal wall
laryng(o)	larynx
lateral	to the side
lateral plane	Imaginary line that divides the body perpendicularly to the medial plane.
left lower quadrant (LLQ)	Quadrant on the lower left anterior side of the patient's body.
left upper quadrant (LUQ)	Quadrant on the upper left anterior side of the patient's body.
linguo	tongue
lip(o)	fat
lumbar region	Left and right regions of the body near the waist on the dorsal (or posterior) side.
lymph(o)	lymph
lymphatic and immune system	Body system that includes the lymph, glands of the lymphatic system, lymphatic vessels, and the specific and nonspecific defenses of the immune system.
mast(o)	breast
maxill(o)	maxilla
medial	At or near the middle (of the body)
medial plane	Imaginary line that divides the body into equal left and right halves.
medull(o)	medulla
mening(o)	meninges
midsagittal plane	See medial plane
muco	mucus
muscle tissue	Tissue that is able to contract and relax
musculoskeletal system	Body system that includes muscles, bones, and cartilage.
my(o)	muscle
myel(o)	spinal cords; bone marrow
nephr(o)	kidney
nervous system	Body system that includes the brain, spinal cord, and nerves and controls most body functions by sending and receiving messages.
nervous tissue	Specialized tissue that forms nerve cells and is capable of transmitting messages.
neur, neuro	nerve
oculo	eye
odont(o)	tooth
onych(o)	nail
oo	egg
oophor(o)	ovary
ophthalm(o	eye
opto, optico	eye; sight

or(o)	mouth
orchi(o), orchid(o)	testis
organ	Group of specialized tissue that performs a specific function.
osseo, ossi	bone
ost(e), osteo	bone
ot(o)	ear
ovari(o)	ovary
ovi, ovo	egg; ova
ped(o), pedi	food; child
pelvi(o), pelvo	pelvic bone; hip
pelvic cavity	Body space below the abdominal cavity that includes the reproductive organs.
pharyng(o)	pharynx
phleb(o)	vein
phren(o), phreni, phrenico	mind; diaphragm
pil(o)	hair
plasma, plasmo, plasmat(o)	plasma
pleur(o), pleura	rib; side; pleura
pneum(a), pneumat(o)	lungs; air; breathing
pod(o)	foot
posterior	At or toward the back side (of the body)
proct(o)	anus
prone	Lying on the stomach with the face down.
proximal	At or near the point of attachment of the trunk.
psych(o), psyche	mind
pulmon(o)	lung
pyel(o)	renal pelvis
rachi(o)	spine
rect(o)	rectum
reni, reno	kidney
reproductive system	Either the male or female body system that controls reproduction
respiratory system	Body system that includes the lings and airways and performs breathing.
rhin(o)	nose
right lower quadrant (RLQ)	Quadrant on the lower right anterior side of the patient's body
right upper quadrant (RUQ)	Quadrant on the upper right anterior side of the patient's body.
sacr(o)	sacrum
sagittal plane	Imaginary line that divides the body into right and left portions.
sarco	fleshy tissue; muscle
scler(o)	sclera
sensory system	Body system that includes the eyes and ears and those parts of other systems involved in the reactions of the five senses.
sial(o)	salivary glands; saliva
sigmoid(o)	sigmoid colon
somat(o)	body

sperma, spermato, spermo	semen; spermatozoa
spinal cavity	Body space that contains the spinal cord.
splanchn(o), splanchni	viscera
splen(o)	spleen
spondyl(o)	vertebra
stern(o)	sternum
steth(o)	chest
stom(a), stomat(o)	mouth
superficial	at or near the surface (of the body).
superior	above another body structure
supine	lying on the spine facing upward.
system	Any group of organs and ancillary parts that work together to perform a major body function.
ten(o), tendin(o), tendo, tenon(o)	tendon
test(o)	testis
thorac(o), thoracico	thorax, chest
thoracic cavity	Body space above the abdominal cavity that contains the heart, lungs, and major blood vessels.
thym(o)	thymus gland
thyr(o)	thyroid gland
tissue	Any group of cells that work together to perform a single function.
trache(o)	trachea
trachel(o)	neck
transverse plane	Imaginary line that intersects the body horizontally.
trich(o), trichi	hair
umbilical region	Area of the body surrounding the umbilicus.
urinary system	Body system that includes the kidneys, ureters, bladder, and urethra and helps maintain homeostasis by removing fluid and dissolved waste.
varico	varicosity
vas(o)	blood vessel; duct
vasculo	blood vessel
veni, veno	vein
ventral	at or toward the front (of the body)
ventral cavity	Major cavity in the front of the body containing the thoracic, abdominal, and pelvic cavities.
ventricul(o)	ventricle
vertebro	vertebra
vesic(o)	bladder
abscess	Localized collection of pus and other exudate, usually accompanied by swelling and redness.
acne	Inflammatory eruption of the skin, occurring in or near sebaceous glands on the face, neck, shoulder, or upper neck.
acne vulgaris	See acne
actinic keratosis	Overgrowth of horny skin that forms from overexposure to sunlight; sunburn.
adip(o)	fatty
adipose	Fatty; relating to fat
allograft	Skin graft using donor skin from one person to another

albinism	Rare, congenital condition causing either partial or total lack of pigmentation.
alopecia areata	Loss of hair in patches, loss of hair in spots, baldness.
alpha-hydroxy acid	Agent added to cosmetics to improve the skin's appearance.
anesthetic	Agent that relieves pain by blocking nerve sensations
antibacterial	Agent that kills or slows the growth of a bacteria.
antibiotic	Agent that kills or slows the growth of microorganisms.
antifungal	Agent that kills or slows the growth of fungi.
antihistamine	Agent that controls allergic reactions by blocking the effectiveness of histamines in the body.
anti-inflammatory	Agent that relieves the symptoms of inflammations.
antipruritic	Agent that controls itching
antiseptic	Agent that kills or slows the growth of microorganisms.
apocrine glands	Glands that appear during and after puberty and secret sweat, as from the armpits.
astringent	Agent that removes excess oils and impurities from the surface of skin.
autograft	Skin graft using skin from one's own body
basal cell carcinoma	Slow-growing cancer of the basal cells of teh epidermis, usually a result of sun damage.
biopsy	Excision of tissue for microscopic examination.
birthmark	Lesion (especially a hemangioma) visible at or soon after birth; nevus
blackhead	See Comedo Open hair follicle filled with bacteria and sebum; common in acne; blackhead.
bulla(pl.bullae)	Bubble-like blister on the surface of the skin.
burn	Damage to the skin caused by exposure to heat, chemicals, electricity, radiation, or other skin irritants.
callus	Mass of hard skin that forms as a cover over broken skin on certain areas of the body, especially the feet and hands.
candidiasis	Yeast-like fungus on the skin, caused by Candida; characterized by pruritus, white exudate, peeling, and easy bleeding; examples are thrush and diaper rash.
carbuncle	Infected area of the skin producing pus and usually accompanied by fever.
cauterize	To apply heat to an area to cause coagulation and stop bleeding.
cellulitis	Severe inflammation of the dermis and subcutaneous portions of the skin, usually caused by an infection that enters the skin through an opening as a wound; characterized by local heat, redness, pain, and swelling.
chemotherapy	Treatment of cancer that uses chemicals to destroy malignant cells
chloasma	Group of fairly large, pigmented facial patches, often associated with pregnancy
cicatrix	Growth of fibrous tissue inside a wound that forms a scar; also, general term for scar.
cold sore	Eruption around the mouth or lips; herpes simplex virus type 1.
collagen	Major protein substance that is tough and flexible and that forms connective tissue in the body.
comedo	Open hair follicle filled with bacteria and sebum; common in acne; blackhead.
corium	See dermis Layer of skin beneath the epidermis containing blood vessels, nerves, and some glands
corn	Growth of hard skin, usually on the toes.
corticosteroid	Agent with anti-inflammatory properties.
crust	Hard layer, especially one found by dried pus, as in a scab.
cryosurgery	Surgery that removes tissue by freezing it with liquid nitrogen.
currettage	Removal of tissue from an area, such as a wound, by scraping.

cuticle	Thin band of epidermis that surrounds the edge of nails, except at the top.
cyst	Abnormal sac containing fluid
debridement	Removal of dead tissue from a wound.
decubitus ulcer	Chronic ulcer on skin over bony parts that are under constant pressure.
depigmentation	Loss of color of the skin
dermabrasion	Removal of wrinkles, scars, tattoos, and other marks by scraping with brushes or emery papers
dermatitis	Inflammation of the skin
dermat(o)	skin
diaphoresis	Excretion of fluid by the sweat glands; sweating.
discord lupus erythematosus	Mild form of lupus
ecchymosis (pl. ecchymoses)	Purplish skin patch(bruise) caused by broken blood vessels beneath the surface.
eccrine glands	sweat glands that occur all over the body, except where the apocrine glands occur.
eczema	severe inflammatory condition of the skin, usually of unknown cause.
electrodesiccation	Drying with electrical current.
emollient	Agent that smooths or softens skin.
epidermis	Outer portion of the skin containing several strata
erosion	wearing away of the surface of the skin, especially that caused by friction.
exanthematous viral disease	Viral disease that causes a rash on the skin.
excoriation	Injury to the surface of the skin caused by a scratch, abrasion, or burn, usually accompanied by some oozing.
exocrine glands	glands that secret through ducts toward the outside of the body
exudate	Any fluid excreted out of tissue, especially fluid excreted out of an injury to the skin.
fever blister	eruption around the mouth or lips; herpes simplex virus Type 1
first-degree burn	least severe burn, causes injury to the surfaces of the skin without blistering.
fissure	Deep slit in the skin.
fulguration	destruction of tissue using electric sparks.
furuncle	localized skin infection, usually in a hair follicle and containing pus; boil
gangrene	Death of an area of skin, usually caused by loss of blood supply to the area.
genital herpes	See herpes simplex virus Type 2 Herpes that recurs on the genitalia; can be easily transmitted from on person to another through sexual contact.
hair follicle	tube-like sac in the epidermis out of which the hair shaft develops.
hair root	portion of hair beneath the skin surface.
hair shaft	portion of the hair visible above the skin surface.
herpes	an inflammatory skin disease caused by viruses of the family Herpesviridae.
herpes simplex virus Type 1	Herpes that recurs on the lips and around the area of the mouth, usually during viral illnesses or states of stress.
herpes simplex virus Type 2	Herpes that recurs on the genitalia; can be easily transmitted from one person to another through sexual contact.
herpes zoster	Painful herpes that affects nerve roots; shingles.
heterograft	skin graft using donor skin from one species to another
hidr(o)	sweat, sweat glands
hives	See urticaria group of reddish wheals, usually accompanied by pruritus and often caused by an allergy.

homograft	skin graft using donor skin from one person to another.
hypodermis	Subcutaneous skin layer; layer below the dermis
ichthy(o)	fish, scaly
impetigo	a type of pyoderma
integument	skin and all the elements that are contained within and arise from it
intradermal	from within the skin, particularly from the dermis
Kaposi's sarcoma	skin cancer associated with AIDS
keloid	thick scarring of the skin that forms after an injury or surgery.
keratin	hard, horny protein that forms nails and hair.
kerat(o)	horny tissue
keratolytic	Agent that aids in the removal of warts and corns.
keratosis	lesion on the epidermis containing keratin
lesion	wound, damage, or injury to the skin.
leukoderma	absence of pigment in the skin or in an area of the skin
leukoplakia	white patch of mucus membrane on the tongue or cheek
lip(o)	fatty
lunula(pl. lunulae)	half-moon shaped area at the base of the nail plate.
macule	small, flat, noticeably colored spot on the skin.
malignant melanoma	virulent skin cancer originating in the melanocytes, usually caused by overexposure to the sun.
Mantoux test	test for tuberculosis in which a small dose of tuberculin in injected into the skin with a syringe.
melan(o)	black, very dark
melanin	pigment produced by melanocytes that determines skin, hair, and eye color.
melanocyte	cell in the epidermis that produces melanin
Moh's surgery	removal of thin layers of malignant tissue until nonmalignant tissues is found.
myc(o)	fungus
nail	thin layer of keratin that covers the distal portion of fingers and toes.
neoplasm	abnormal tissue growth.
nevus(pl. nevi)	birthmark
nodule	small knob of tissue
onych(o)	nail
onychia, onychitis	inflammation of the nail
onychopathy	disease of the nail.
papillary layer	thin sublayer of the dermis containing small papillae (nipple-like masses).
papule	small, solid elevation on the skin
parasiticide	Agent that kills or slows the growth of parasites.
paronychia	inflammation, with pus, of the fold surrounding the nail plate.
patch	small area of skin differing in color from the surrounding area.
patch test	test for allergic sensitivity in which a small dose of antigen is applied to the skin on a small piece of gauze
pediculated polyp	polyp that projects upward from slender stalk.
pediculosis	lice infestation
pemphigus	autoimmune disease that causes skin blistering
petechia(pl. petechiae)	tiny hemorrhages beneath the surface of the skin.
pil(o)	hair
pilonidal cyst	cyst containing hair, usually found at the lower end of the spinal cord.

plantar wart	wart on the sole of the foot.
plaque	see patch small area of skin differing in color from the surrounding area.
plastic surgery	repair or reconstruction(as of the skin) by means of surgery.
polyp	bulging mass of tissue that projects outward from the skin surface.
pore	opening or hole, particularly in the skin.
pressure sore	See decubitus ulcer. Chronic ulcer on skin over bony parts that are under constant pressure.
pruritus	itching
psoriasis	chronic skin condition accompanied by scaly lesions with extreme pruritus.
purpura	skin condition with extensive hemorrhages underneath the skin covering a wide area.
pustule	small elevation on the skin containing pus.
pyoderma	any inflammation of the skin that produces pus.
radiation therapy	treatment of cancer that uses ionizing radiation to destroy malignant cells.
reticular layer	Bottom sublayer of the dermis containing reticula(network of structures with connective tissue between).
ringworm	fungal infection; tinea
rosacea	vascular disease that causes blotchy, red patches on the skin, particularly on the nose and cheeks.
roseola	skin eruption small, rosy patches, usually caused by a virus.
rubella	disease that causes a viral skin rash; German measles.
rubeola	disease that causes a viral skin rash; measles.
scabies	skin eruption caused by a mite burrowing into the skin.
scale	small plate of hard skin that falls off.
Schick test	test for diphtheria
scleroderma	thickening of the skin caused by an increase in collagen formation.
scratch test	test for allergic sensitivity in which a small amount of antigen is scratched onto the surface of the skin.
sebaceous cyst	cyst containing yellow sebum.
sebaceous glands	glands in the dermis that open to hair follicles and secrete sebum.
seb(o)	sebum, sebaceous glands.
seborrhea	overproduction of sebum by the sebaceous glands.
sebum	oily substance, usually secreted into hair follicle.
second-degree burn	moderately severe burn that affects the epidermis and dermis; usually involves blistering.
sessile polyp	polyp that projects upward from a broad base.
shingles	viral disease affecting peripheral nerves and caused by herpes zoster.
skin graft	placement of fresh skin over a damaged area.
squamous cell carcinoma	cancer of the squamous epithelium
squamous epithelium	flat, scaly layer of cells that makes up the epidermis.
steat(o)	fat
stratified squamous epithelium	layers of epithelial cells that make up the strata of the epidermis.
stratum(pl. strata)	layer of tissue, especially a layer of skin.
striae	stretch marks made in the collagen fibers of the dermis layer.
subcutaneous layer	bottom layer of the skin containing fatty tissue.
sweat glands	coiled glands of the skin that secrete perspiration to regulate body temperature and excrete waste products.

systemic lupus erythematosus	most severe form of lupus, involving internal organs.
third-degree burns	most severe type of burns; involving complete destruction of an area of skin.
tine test	test for tuberculosis in which a small dose of tuberculin is injected into a series of sites within a small space with a tine (instrument that punctures the surface of the skin).
tinea	fungal infection; ringworm
topical anesthetic	anesthetic applied to the surface of the skin.
trich(o)	hair
tumor	any mass of tissue; swelling
ulcer	open lesion, usually with superficial loss of tissue.
ultraviolet light	artificial sunlight used to treat some skin lesions.
urticaria	group of reddish wheals, usually accompanied by pruritus and often caused by an allergy.
varicella	contagious skin disease, usually occurring during childhood, often accompanied by the formation of pustules; chicken pox.
vascular lesion	lesion in a blood vessel that shows through the skin.
verruca (pl. verrucae)	flesh-colored growth, sometimes caused by a virus; wart.
vesicle	small, raised sac on the skin containing fluid.
vitiligo	condition in which white patches appear on otherwise normally pigmented skin.
wart	See verruca flesh-colored growth, sometimes caused by virus; wart
wheal	itchy patch of raised skin.
whitehead	closed comedo that does not contain the dark bacteria present in blackheads.
xanth(o)	yellow
xenograft	See heterograft skin graft using donor skin from species to another.
xer(o)	dry
bx	biopsy
DLE	Discoid Lupus Erythematosus
PPD	Psoralen-ultraviolet a light therapy
SLE	System Lupus Erythematosus
acetabul(o)	acetabulum
acetabulum	cup-shaped depression in the hip bone into which the top of the femur fits.
acromi(o)	end point of the scapula
acromion	part of the scapula that connects to the clavicle.
amphiarthroses	cartilaginous joint having some movement at the union of two bones
amputation	Cutting off of a limb or part of a limb.
analgesic	to relieve pain aspirin acetaminophen (NSAIDS are also analgesics.) Agents that relieve pain.
ankle	Hinged area between the lower leg bones and the bones of the foot.
ankyl(o)	bent crooked
ankylosis	Stiffing of a joint, especially as a result of disease.
anti-inflammatory	Agent that reduces inflammation.
arthr(o)	joint
arthaglgia	Severe joint pain
arthritis	Any of various conditions involving joint inflammation.
arthrocentesis	removal of fluid from a joint with use of puncture needle.
arthrodesis	Surgical fusion of a joint to stiffen it

arthography	Radiography of a joint
arthroplasty	Surgical replacement or repair of a joint.
arthroscopy	Examination with an instrument that explores the interior of a joint.
articular cartilage	cartilage joint
articulation	point at which two bones join together to allow movement.
atlas	First cervical vertebra
atrophy	Wasting away of tissue, organs, and cells, usually as a result of disease or loss of blood supply.
axis	second cervical vertebra.
bone	Hard connective tissue that forms the skeleton of the body.
bone grafting	Transplantation of bone from one site to another.
bone head	Upper, rounded end of a bone.
bone phagocyte	Bone cell that ingests dead bone and bone debris
bone scan	radiographic or ultrasound image of a bone.
bony necrosis	death of portions of bone.
brachi(o)	arm
bunion	an inflamed bursa at the foot joint, between the big toe and the first metatarsal bone.
bunionectomy	removal of a bunion
burs(o)	bursa
bursa	sac lined with a synovail membrane that fills the spaces between tendons and joints.
bursectomy	removal of a bursa
bursitis	inflammation of bursa
calcane(o)	heel
calcaneus	heel bone
calcar	another name for spur
calci(o)	calcium
calcium	Mineral important in the formation of bone.
cancellous bone	Spongy bone with latticelike structure.
cardiac muscle	Striated involuntary muscle of the heart.
carp(o)	wrist
carpal tunnel syndrome	pain and paraesthesia in the hand due to repetitive motion injury of the median nerve.
carpus, carpal bone	wrist bone
cartilage	flexible connective tissue found in joints, fetal skeleton, and the lining of various parts of the body.
cartilaginous disk	Thin, circular mass of cartilage between the vertebrae of the spinal column.
casting	forming of a cast in a mold; placing of fiberglass or plaster over a body part to prevent its movement.
cephal(o)	head
cervic(o)	neck
cervical vertebrae	Seven vertebrae of the spinal column located in the neck.
chiropractor	Health care professional who works to align the spinal column so as to treat certain ailments
chondr(o)	cartilage
chondromalacia	softening of cartilage
clavicle	curved bone of the shoulder that joins to the scapula; collar bone.

closed fracture	fracture with no open skin wound.
coccyx	small bone consisting of four fused vertebrae at the end of the spinal column; tailbone
Colles' fracture	fracture of lower end of the radius.
comminuted fracture	fracture with shattered bones.
compact bone	hard bone with tightly woven structure.
complex fracture	fracture with part of the bone displaced.
compound fracture	fracture with an open skin wound; open fracture.
compression fracture	fracture of one or more vertebrae caused by compressing on the space between the vertebrae.
condyle(o)	knob, knuckle
cost(o)	rib
crani(o)	skull
crest	bony ridge
dactyl(o)	fingers, toes
degenerative arthritis	arthritis with erosion of the cartilage.
densitometer	device that measures bone density using light and x-rays.
diaphysis	long middle section of a long bone; shaft
diarthroses	freely movable joints.
disk, disc(disk)	thin, circular mass of cartilage between the vertebrae of the spinal column.
diskography	radiographic image of intervertebral disk by injection of a contrast medium into the center of the disk.
dislocation	movement of a joint out of its normal position as a result of an injury or sudden, strenuous movement.
dorsal vertebrae	thoracic vertebrae
dystonia	abnormal tone in the tissues
elbow	joint between the upper arm and the forearm.
electromyogram	a graphic image of muscular action using electrical currents
endosteum	lining of the medullary cavity
epiphyseal plate	cartilaginous tissue that is replaced during growth years, but eventually calcifies and disappears when growth stops.
epiphysitis	inflammation of the epiphysis.
ethmoid bone	irregular bone of the face attached to the sphenoid bone.
ethmoid sinuses	sinuses on both sides of the nasal cavities between each eye and the sphenoid sinus.
exostosis	abnormal bone growth capped with cartilage.
external fixation device	device applied externally to hold a limb in place.
fasci(o)	fascia
fascia	sheet pf fibrous tissue that encloses muscles
femor(o)	femur
femur	long bone of the thigh.
fibr(o)	fiber
fibula	smallest long bone of the lower leg.
fissure	deep furrow or slit.
flaccid	without tone; relaxed
flat bone	thin, flattened bones that cover certain areas, as of the skull.
fontanelle	soft, membranous section on top of an infant's skull.
formen	opening or perforation through a bone.

formen magnum	opening in the occipital bone through which the spinal cord passes.
fossa	depression, as in a bone.
fracture	a break, especially in a bone.
frontal bone	large bone of the skull that forms the top of the head and forehead.
frontal sinuses	sinuses above the eyes.
goniometer	instrument that measures angles or range of motion in a joint.
gouty arthritis, gout	inflammation of the joints, present in gout; usually caused by uric acid crystals.
greenstick fracture	fracture with twisting or bending of the bone but no breaking; usually occurs in children.
hairline fracture	fracture with no bone separation or fragmentation.
heel	back, rounded portion of the foot.
herniated disk	protrusion of an intervertebral disk into neural canal
humer(o)	humerus
humerus	long bone of the arm connecting to the scapula on top and the radius and ulna at the bottom.
hypertrophy	abnormal increase as in muscle size.
hypotonia	abnormally reduced muscle tension,
ilo(o)	ilium
ilium	wide portion of the hip bone.
impacted fracture	fracture in which a fragment from on part of the fracture is driven into the tissue of another part.
imcomplete fracture	fracture that does not go entirely through a bone.
insertion	point at which muscles attach to a movable bone.
internal fixation device	device, such as a pin, inserted in bone to hold it in place.
involuntary muscle	muscles not movable at will.
irregular bones	any of a group of bones with a special shape to fit into certain area of the skeleton, such as the skull.
ischi(o)	ischium
ischium	one of three fused bones that form the pelvic girdle.
joint	place of joining between two or more bones.
kyph(o)	hump, bent
kyphosis	abnormal posterior spine curvature.
lacrimal bone	thin, flat bone of the face.
lamin(o)	lamina
lamina, (pl. laminae)	thin, flat part of either side of the arch of a vertebra.
laminectomy	removal of part of an invertebral disk.
leiomy(o)	smooth muscle
leiomyoma	benign tumor of smooth muscle.
leiomyosarcoma	malignant tumor of smooth muscle.
ligament	sheet of fibrous tissue connecting and supporting bones; attaches bone to bone.
long bone	any bone of the extremities with a shaft.
lordosis	abnormal anterior spine curvature resulting in a sway back.
lumb(o)	lumbar
lumbar vertebrae	five vertebrae of the lower back.
malleolus (pl. malleoli)	rounded protrusion of the tibia of fibula on either side of the ankle.
mandible	U-shaped bone of the lower jaw
mandibular bone	mandible.

marrow	connective tissue filling the medullary cavity, often rich in nutrients.
mastoid process	protrusion of the temporal bone that sits behind the ear.
maxill(o)	upper jaw
maxillary bone	bone of the upper jaw
maxillary sinus	sinus on either side of the nasal cavity below the eyes.
medullary cavity	soft center cavity in bone that often holds marrow.
metacarp(o)	metacarpal
metacarpal	one of the five bones of the hand between the wrist and the fingers.
metaphysis	section of long bone between the epiphysis and diaphysis.
metatarsal bones	bones of the foot between the instep(arch) and the toes.
muscle	contractile tissue that plays a major role in body movement.
muscle relaxant	agent that relieves muscle stiffness.
muscular dystrophy	progressive degenerative disorder affecting the musculoskeletal system, and later, other organs.
musculoskeletal system	system of the body including the muscles and skeleton.
my(o)	muscle
myalgia	muscle pain
myel(o)	spinal cord; bone marrow
myelography	radiographic imaging of the spinal cord
myeloma	bone marrow
myodynia	muscle pain
myoma	benign muscle tumor
myoplasty	surgical repair of muscle tissue
myositis	inflammation of a muscle.
narcotic	agent that relieves pain by affecting the body in ways similar to opium.
nasal bones	bones that form the bridge of the nose
nasal cavity	cavity on either side of the nasal septum.
neural canal	space through which the spinal cord passes.
nonsteriodal anti-inflammatory drug	agent that reduces inflammation without the use of steroids.
nucleus pulposus	fibrous mass in the center portion of the intervertebral disk.
occipital bone	bone that forms the lower back portion of the skull
olecranon	curved end of the ulna to which tendons of the arm muscles attach; bony prominence of the elbow.
open fracture	fracture with an open skin wound; compound fracture.
origin	point at which muscles attach to stationary bone.
orthopedist	physician who examines, diagnoses, and treats disorders of the musculoskeletal system.
orthosis, orthotic	external appliance used to immobilize or assist the movement of the spine or limbs.
osseus tissue	connective tissue into which calcium salts are deposited.
ossification	hardening into bone.
oste(o)	bone
osteaglia	bone pain
osteoarthritis	arthritis with loss of cartilage.
osteoblast	cells that forms bone.
osteoclasis	breaking of a bone in order to repair or reposition it.
osteoclast	large cells that reabsorbs and removes osseous tissue.

osteocyte	bone cell
osteodynia	bone pain
osteoma	benign tumor, usually in the skull or mandible.
osteomyelitis	inflammation of the bone marrow and surrounding bone.
osteopath	physician who combines manipulative treatment with conventional therapeutic measures.
osteoplasty	surgical replacement or repair of bone.
osteoporosis	degenerative thinning of bone.
osteoscarcoma	malignant tumor of bone.
osteotomy	cutting of bone.
palatine bone	bones that help form the hard palate and nasal cavity; located behind the maxillary bones.
parietal bone	flat, curved bone either side of the upper part of the skull.
patall(o)	knee
patella	large, sesamoid bone that forms the kneecap
pathological fracture	fracture occurring at the site of already damaged bone.
ped(i), pedo	foot
pelvi(o)	pelvis
pelvic cavity	cup-shaped cavity formed by the large bones of the pelvic girdle; contains female reproductive organs, sigmoid colon, bladder, and rectum.
pelvic girdle	hip bones.
pelvis	cup-shaped ring of bone and ligaments at the base of the trunk.
periosteum	fibrous membrane covering the surface of bone.
phalang(o)	finger or toe bone
phanlanges (sing. phalanx)	long bones of the fingers and toes.
phantom limbs; phantom pain	pain felt in a paralyzed or amputated limb.
phosphorus	mineral important to the formation of bone.
physical therapy	movement therapy to restore use of damaged areas of the body.
pod(o)	foot
podagra	pain in the big toe, often associated with gout.
podiatrist	medical specialist who examines, diagnoses, and treats disorders if the foot.
process	bony outgrowth or projection.
prosthetic device	artificial device used as a substitute for a missing or diseased body part.
pub(o)	pubis
pubes	anteroinferior portion of the hip bone.
pubic symphysis	joint between the two pubic bones.
rachi(o)	spine
radi(o)	forearm bone
radius	shorter bone of the forearm.
reduction	return of a part to its normal position.
rhabd(o)	rod-shaped
rhabdomy(o)	striated muscle
rhabdomyoma	benign tumor in striated muscle.
rhabdomyosarcoma	malignant tumor in striated muscle.
rheumatoid arthritis	autoimmune disorder affecting connective tissue.

rheumatoid factor test	test used to detect rheumatoid arthritis
rhematologist	physician who examines, diagnoses, and treats disorders of the joints and musculoskeletal system.
rib	one of twenty-four bones that form the chest wall.
rickets.	disease of the skeletal system, usually caused by vitamin d deficiency.
rigidity	stiffness
rigor	stiffening
sacrum	next-to-last spinal vertebra made up of five fused bones; vertebra that forms part of the pelvis.
scapul(o)	scapula
scapula	large flat bone that forms the shoulder blade.
sciatica	pain in the lower back, usually radiating down the leg, from a herniated disk or other injury or condition.
scoli(o)	curved
scoliosis	abnormal lateral curvature of the spinal column.
sella turcica	bony depression in the sphenoid bone where the pituitary gland is located
sequestrum	piece of dead tissue or bone separated from the surrounding area.
serum calcium	test for calcium in the blood.
serum creatine phosphokinase	enzyme active in muscle contraction, usually elevated after a myocardial infarction and in the presence of other degenerative muscle disease.
serum phosphorus	test for phosphorus in the blood.
sesamoid bone	bone formed in a tendon over a joint.
shin	anterior ridge of the tibia.
short bones	square-shaped bones with approximately equal dimensions on all sides.
simple fracture	fracture with no open skin wound.
sinus	hollow cavity, especially either side of two cavities on the sides of the nose.
skeleton	bony framework of the body.
smooth muscle	fibrous muscle of internal organs that acts involuntarily.
spasm	sudden, involuntary muscle contraction.
spactic	tending to have spasms.
sphenoid bone	bone that forms the base of the skull
sphenoid sinus	sinus above and behind the nose
spina bifida	congenital defect with deformity of the spinal column.
spinal column	column of vertebrae at the posterior of the body, from the neck to the coccyx.
spinal curvature	abnormal curvature of the spine.
spinous process	protrusion from the center of the vertebral arch.
splinting	applying a splint to immobilize a body part.
spondyl(o)	vertebra
spondylolisthesis	degenerative condition in which one vertebra misaligns with the one below it.
spondylolysis	degenerative condition of the moving part of a vertebra.
spondylosndesis	fusion of two or more spinal vertebrae.
spongy bone	bone with an open latticework filled with connective tissue or marrow.
sprain	injury to a joint without dislocation or fracture.
spur	bony projection growing out of a bone.
stern(o)	sternum
strain	injury to a muscle as a result of overuse.
striated muscle	muscle with a ribbed appearance that is controlled at will.

styloid process	peg-shaped protrusion from a bone.
subluxation	partial dislocation, as between joint surfaces.
sulcus	groove or furrow in the surface of bone.
suture	joining of two bones parts with fibrous membrane
symphysis	type of cartilaginous joint uniting two bones.
synarthrosis	fibrous joint with no movement.
synov(o)	synovial membrane
synovectomy	removal of part or all of a joint's synovial membrane.
synovial fluid	fluid that serves to lubricate joints.
synovial joint	a joint that moves
synovial membrane	connective tissue lining the cavity of joints and producing the synovial fluid.
talipes calcaneus	deformity of the heel resulting from weakened calf muscles.
talipes valgus	foot deformity characterized by eversion of the foot
talipes varus	foot deformity characterized by inversion of the foot.
tars(o)	tarsus
tarsus, tarsal bones	seven bones of the instep (arch of the foot)
temporal bone	large bone forming the base and sides if the skull
temporomandibular joint	joint of the lower jaw between the temporal bone and the mandible.
ten(o), tend(o), tendin(o)	tendon
tendinitis, tendonitis	inflammation of a tendon
tendon	fibrous band that connects muscle to bone or other structures.
tenotomy	surgical cutting of a tendon.
tetany	painfully long muscle contraction.
thorac(o)	thorax
thoracic vertebrae	twelve vertebrae of the chest area.
tibi(o)	tibia
tibia	larger of the two lower leg bones
tinel's sign	"pins and needles" sensation felt when an injured nerve site is trapped.
traction	dragging or pulling or straightening of something, as a limb, by attachment of elastic or other devices.
transverse process	protrusion on either side of the vertebral arch.
tremor	abnormal, repetitive muscle contractions.
trochanter	bony protrusion at the upper end of the femur.
true rib	seven upper ribs of the chest that attach to the sternum.
tubercle	slight bony elevation to which a ligament or muscle may be attached.
tuberosity	larger elevation in the surface of a bone.
uln(o)	ulna
ulna	larger bone of the forearm
uric acid test	test for acid content in urine, elevated levels may indicate gout.
vertebr(o)	vertebra
vertebra (pl. vertebrae)	one of the bony segments of the spinal column.
vertebral body	main portion of the vertebra, separated from arches of the vertebra
vertebral column	spinal column
visceral muscle	smooth muscle
vitamin d	vitamin important to the formation of bone
voluntary muscle	striated muscle
vomer	flat bone forming the nasal septum

zygomatic bone	bone that forms the cheek
A-K	above the knee (amputation)
B-K	below the knee (amputation)
C1, C2, etc.	first cervical vertebra, second cervical vertebra, etc.
ca	calcium
CTS	carpal tunnel syndrome
DJD	degenerative joint disease
DTR	deep tendon reflux
EMG	electromyogram
fx	fracture
IM	intramuscularly
L1, L2, etc.	first lumbar vertebra, second lumbar vertebra, etc.
MCP	metacarpophalangeal
NSAID	nonsteroidal anti-inflammatory drug
P	phosphorus
PIP	proximal interphalangeal joint
ROM	range of motion
T1, T2, etc.	first thoracic vertebra, second thoracic vertebra, etc.
TMJ	temporomandibular joint.
anastomosis	surgical connection of two blood vessels to allow blood flow between them.
aneurysm	ballooning of the artery wall caused by weakness in the wall.
angina	angina pectoris
angina pectoris	chest pain, usually caused by a lowered oxygen or blood supply to the heart.
angi(o)	blood vessel
angiocardiography	viewing of the heart and its major blood vessel by x-ray after injection of a contrast medium.
angiography	viewing of the heart's major blood vessels by x-ray after injection of a contrast medium.
angioplasty	opening of a blocked blood vessel, as by balloon dilation.
angioscopy	viewing of the interior of a blood vessel using a fiberoptic catheter inserted or threaded into the vessel
angiotensin converting enzyme inhibitor	medication used for heart failure and other cardiovascular problems; acts by dilating arteries to lower blood pressure and makes heart pump easier.
antianginal	agent used to relieve or prevent attacks of angina
antiarrhythmic	agent used to help normalize cardiac rhythm
anticlotting	agent that prevents the formation of dangerous clots.
anticoagulant	agent that prevents the formation of dangerous clots.
antihypertensive	agent that helps control high blood pressure
aorta	largest artery of the body; artery through which blood exits the heart.
aort(O)	aorta
aortic regurgitation or reflux	backward flow or leakage of blood through a faulty aortic valve.
aortic valve	valve between the aorta and the left ventricle.
aortography	viewing of the aorta by x-ray after injection of contrast medium.
arrhythmia	irregularity in the rhythm of the heartbeat.
arteri(o) arter(o)	artery
arteriography	viewing of a specific artery by x-ray after injection of contrast medium
arteriole	a tiny artery connecting to a capillary.

arteriosclerosis	hardening of the arteries.
arteriotomy	surgical incision into an artery, especially to remove a clot.
arteritis	inflammation of an artery or arteries.
artery	a thick-walled blood vessel that, in systemic circulation, carries oxygenated blood away from the heart.
asystole	cardiac arrest
ather(o)	fatty matter
atherectomy	surgical removal of an atheroma
atheroma	a fatty deposit (plaque) in the wall of an artery.
atherosclerosis	hardening of the arteries caused by the building of atheromas
atri(o)	atrium
atrial fibrillation	an irregular, usually rapid, heartbeat caused by overstimulation of the AV node.
atrioventricular block	heart block; partial or complete blockage of the electrical impulses from the atrioventricular node.
atrioventricular bundle	bundles of fibers in the interventricular septum that transfer charges in the heart's conduction system; also called bundle of His.
atrioventricular node (AV node)	specialized part of the interatrail septum that sends a charge to the bundle of His.
atrioventricular valve	one of two valves that control blood flow between the atria and ventricles.
atrium (pl. atria)	either of the two upper chambers of the heart.
auscultation	process of listening to body sounds via a stethoscope.
bacterial endocarditis	bacterial inflammation of the inner lining of the heart.
balloon catheter dilation	insertion of a balloon catheter into a blood vessel to open the passage so blood can flow freely
balloon valvuloplasty	procedure that uses a balloon catheter to open narrowed orifices in cardiac valves.
bicuspid valve	atrioventricular valve on the left side of the heart.
blood	essential fluid containing plasma and other elements that circulates throughout the body; delivers nutrients to and removes waste from the body's cells.
blood pressure	measure of the force of blood surging against the walls of the arteries.
blood vessel	any of the tubular passageways in the cardiovascular systems through which blood travels.
bradycardia	heart rate of fewer than 60 beats per minute.
bruit	sound of murmur, especially an abnormal heart sound heard on auscultation, especially of the carotid artery.
bundle of His	bundle of fibers in the interventricular septum that transfer charges in the heart's conduction system
bypass	a structure (usually a vein graft) that creates a new passage for blood to flow from one artery to another artery or part of an artery; used to create a detour around blockages in arteries.
calcium channel blocker	medication that lessens the ability of calcium ions to enter heart and blood vessel muscle; used to lower blood pressure and normalize some arrhythmias.
capillary	a tiny blood vessel that forms the exchange point between the arterial and venous vessels.
carbon dioxide	waste material transported in the venous blood
cardi(o)	heart
cardiac arrest	sudden stopping of the heart; also called asystole.
cardiac catheterziation	process of passing a thin catheter through an artery or vein to the heart to take blood samples, inject a contrast medium, or measure various pressures.
cardiac cycle	repeated contraction and relaxation of the heart as it circulates blood within

	itself and pumps it out to the rest of the body or the lungs.
cardiac enzyme studies	blood test for determining levels of enzymes during a myocardial infarction serum enzyme tests.
cardiac MRI	viewing of the heart by magnetic resonance imaging.
cardiac scan	process of viewing the heart muscle at work by scanning the heart of a patient into whom a radioactive substance has been injected.
cardiac tamponade	compression of the heart caused by fluid accumulation in the pericardial sac.
cardiomyopathy	disease of the heart muscle
cardiopulmonary bypass	procedure used during surgery to divert blood flow to and from the heart through a heart-lung machine and back into circulation.
cardiotonic	medication for congestive heart failure; increases the force of contractions of the myocardium.
carotid artery	artery that transport oxygenated blood to the head and neck
cholesterol	fatty substance present in animal fats, cholesterol circulates in the bloodstream, sometimes causing arterial plaque to form.
claudication	limping caused by inadequate blood supply during activity; usually subsides during rest.
coarctation of the aorta	abnormal narrowing of the aorta
conduction system	part of the heart containing specialized tissue that sends charges through heart fibers, causing the heart to contract and relax at regular intervals.
congenital heart disease	heart disease (usually a type of malformation) that exists at birth.
congestive heart failure	inability of the heart to pump enough blood out during the cardiac cycle; collection of fluid in the lungs result.
constriction	compression or narrowing caused by contraction, as of a vessel.
coronary angioplasty	opening of a blocked blood vessel, as by balloon dilation.
coronary artery	blood vessel that supplies oxygen-rich blood to the heart.
coronary artery disease	condition that reduces the flow of blood and nutrients through the arteries of the heart.
coronary bypass surgery	a structure (usually a vein graft) that creates a new passage for blood to flow from one artery to another artery or part of an artery; used to create a detour around blockages in arteries.
cyanosis	bluish or purplish coloration, as of the skin, caused by deficient oxygenation of the blood.
deep vein thrombosis	formation of a thrombus (clot) in a deep vein, such as femoral vein.
depolarization	contracting state if the myocardial tissue in the heart's conduction system.
diastole	relaxation phase of a heartbeat
digital subtraction angiography	use of two angigrams done with different dyes to provide a comparison bewteen the results.
diuretic	medication that promotes the excretion of urine
doppler ultrasound	ultrasound test of blood flow in certain vessels.
ductus arteriosus	structure in the fetal circulatory systems through which blood flows to bypass the fetus's nonfunctioning lungs.
ductus venosus	structure in the fetal circulatory system through which blood flows to bypass the fetal liver.
dysrthythmia	abnormal heart rhythm.
echocardiography	use of sound waves to produce images showing the structure and motion of the heart.
ejection fraction	percentage of teh volume of teh contents of the left ventricle ejected with each contratction.
electrocardiography	use of the electrocardiograph in diagnosis.

embolectomy	surgical removal of an embolus
embolus	mass of foreign materail blocking a vessel.
endarterectomy	surgical removal of the diseased portion of the lining of an artery
endocarditis	inflammation of the endocardium, espcecially one caused by a bacterial, (for example, staphylococci) or fungal agent.
endocardium	membranous lining of the chambers and valves of the heart, the innermost layer of heart tissues.
endothelium	lining of the arteries that secretes substances into the blood.
endovascular surgery	any of various procedures performed during cardiac catheterization, such as angioscopy and atherectomy.
epicardium	outermost layer of the heart tissue.
essentail hypertension	high blood pressure without any known cause
femoral artery	an artery that supplies blood to the thigh.
fibrillation	random, chaotic, irregular heart rthythm.
flutter	regular but very rapid heartbeat.
Fontan's operation	surgical procedure that create's a bypass from the right atrium to the main pulmonary artery; Fontan's procedure.
foramen ovale	opening in the septum of the fetal heart that closes at birth.
gallop	triple sound of a heartbeat, usually indicative of serious heart disease.
graft	any tissue or organ implanted to replace or mend damaged areas.
hardening of the arteries	ateriosclerosis
heart	musclar organ that receives blood from the veins and sends it into the arteries.
heart block	heart block; partial or complete blockage of the electrical impulses from the artrioventricular node to the ventricles.
heart transplant	implantation of the heart of a person who has just died into a person whose diseased heart cannot sustain life.
hemangi(o)	blood vessel
hemorrhoidectomy	surgical removal of hemmorrhoids.
hemorrhoids	varicose condition of veins in the anal region.
heparin	anticoagulant present in the body; also, synthetic version administered to prevent clotting.
high blood pressure	chronic condition with blood pressure greater than 140/90
Holter monitor	portable device that provides a 24-hour electrocardiogram.
hypertension	chronic condition with blood pressure greater than 140/90
hypertension heart disease	heart disease caused, or worsened, by high blood pressure.
hypotension	chronic condition with blood pressure below normal.
infarct	area of necrosis caused by a sudden drop in the supply of arterial or venous blood.
infarction	sudden drop in the supply of arterial or venous blood, often due to an embolus or thrombus.
inferior vena cava	large vein that draws blood from the lower part of the body to the right atrium.
intermittent claudication	attacks of limping, particularly in the legs, due to ischemia of the muscles.
intracardiac tumor	a tumor within one of the heart chambers.
intravascular stent	stent placed within a blood vessel to allow blood to flow freely.
ischemia	localized blood insufficiency caused by an obstruction.
left atrium	upper left heart chamber
left ventricle	lower left heart chamber
lipid-lowering	helpful in lowering cholesterol levels.

lipid profile	laboratory test that provides the levels of lipids, triglycerides, and other substances in the blood.
low blood pressure	chronic condition with blood pressure below normal
lumen	channel inside an artery through which blood flows.
mitral insufficiency or reflux	backward flow of blood due to a damaged mitral valve.
mitral stenosis	abnormal narrowing at the opening of the mitral valve.
mitral valve	atrioventricular valve on the left side of the heart
mitral valve prolapse	backward flow of blood into the left atrium due to protrusion of one or both mitral cusps into the left atrium during contractions.
multiple-gated acquisition angiography (MUGA)	radioactive scan showing heart function
murmur	soft heart humming sound heard between normal beats.
myocardial infarction	sudden drop in the supply of blood to an area of the heart muscle, usually due to a blockage in a coronary artery.
myocarditis	inflammation of the myocardium
necrosis	death of tissue or an organ or part due to irreversible damage; usually a result of oxygen deprivation.
nitrate	any of several medications that dilate the veins, arteries, or coronary arteries; used to control angina.
occlusion	the closing of a blood vessel
pacemaker	term for the sinoatrial node (SA node); also, an artifical device that regulates heart rhythm.
palpitations	uncomfortable pulsations of the heart felt as a thumping in the chest.
patent ductus arteroosus	a condition at birth in which the ductus arteriosus, a small duct between the aorta and the pulmonary artery, remains abnormally open.
percutaneous transluminal coronary angioplasty	insertion of a balloon catheter into a blood vessel to open the passage so blood can flow freely.
perfusion deficit	lack if flow through a blood vessel, usually caused by an occlusion.
pericardi(o)	pericardium
pericarditis	inflammation of the pericardium
pericardium	protective covering of the heart.
peripheral vascular disease	vascular disease in the lower extremities, usually due to blockages in the arteries of the groin or legs.
petechiae	minute hemorrhages in the skin
phleb(o)	vein
phlebitis	inflammation of the vein
phlebography	viewing of a vein by x-ray after injection of a contrast medium.
phlebotomy	drawing blood from a vein via a small incision
plaque	buildup of solid material, such as fatty deposit, on the lining of an artery.
polarization	resting state of the myocardial tissue in the conduction system of the heart.
popliteal artery	an artery that supplies blood to the cells of the area behind the knee.
positron emission tomography scans	type of nuclear image that measures movement of areas of the heart.
premature atrial contractions (PACs)	atrial contractions that occur before normal impulse; can be the cause of palpitations.
premature ventricular contractions (PVCs)	ventricular contractions that occur before the normal impulse; can be the cause of palpitations.

pulmonary artery	one of two arteries that carry blood that is low in oxygen from the heart to the lungs.
pulmonary artery stenosis	narrowing of the pulmonary artery, preventin the lungs from receiving enought blood from the heart to oxygenate.
pulmonary edema	abnormal accumulation of fluid in the lungs
pulmonary valve	valve that controls the blood flow between the right ventricle and the pulmonary arteries.
pulmonary vein	one of four veins that bring oxygenated blood from the lungs to the left atrium.
pulse	rhythmic expansion and contraction of blood vessel, usually an artery.
Purkinje fibers	fibers in the ventricle that cause it to contract.
Raynaud's phenomenon	spasm in the arteries of the fingers causing numbness or pain.
repolarization	recharging state; transiion from contraction to resting that occurs in the conduction system of the heart.
rheumatic heart disease	heart valve and/or muscle damage caused by an untreated streptococcal infection.
right atrium	upper right chamber of the heart
right ventricle	lower right chamber of the heart
risk factor	any of various factors considered to increase the probability that a disease will occur; for example, high blood pressure and smoking are considered risk factors for heart disease.
rub	frictional sound heard between heartbeats, usually indicating a pericardial murmur.
saphenous vein	any group of veins that transport deoxygenated blood from the legs.
secondary hypertension	hypertension having a known cause, such as kidney disease.
semilunar valve	one of the two valves that prevent the backflow of blood flowing out of the heart into the aorta and the pulmonary artery.
septal defect	congenital abnormality consisting of an opening in the septum between the atria or ventricles.
septum	partition between the left and right chambers of the heart
serum enzyme tests	laboratory test performed to detect enzymes present during or after a myocardial infarction; cardiac enzyme studies.
sinoatrial node (SA node)	region of the right atrium containing specialized tissue that sends electrical impulses to the heart muscle; causing it to connect.
sinus rhythm	normal heart rhythm
sonography	production of images based on the echoes of sound waves against structures.
sphygm(o)	pulse
sphygmomanometer	device for measuring blood pressure
stenosis	narrowing, particularly of blood vessel or of the cardiac valves.
stent	surgically implanted device used to hold something (as a blood vessel) open.
stress test	test that measures heart rate, blood pressure, and other body functions while the patient is exercising on a treadmill.
superior vena cava	large vein that transport blood collected from the upper part of the body to the heart.
systole	contraction phase of the heartbeat
tachycardia	heart rate greater than 100 beats per minute.
tetralogy of Fallot	set of four congenital heart abnomralities appearing together that cause deoxygenated blood to enter the systemic circulation; ventricular septal defect, pulmonary stenosis, incorrect position of the aorta, and right ventricular hypertrophy.
thromb(o)	blood clot

thrombectomy	surgical removal of a thrombus
thrombolytic	agent the dissolves a thrombus
thrombophlebitis	inflammation of a vein with a thrombus
thrombosis	presence of a thrombus in a blood vessek.
thrombotic occlusion	narrowing caused by a thrombus.
thrombus	stationary blood clot in the cardiovascular system, usually found from matter found in the blood.
tissue-type plasminogen activator (tPA, TPA)	agent that prevents a thrombus from forming.
tricuspid stenosis	abnormal narrowing of the opening of the tricuspid valve.
triglyceride	fatty substance; lipid
valve	any of various structures that slow or prevent fluid from flowing backward or forward
valve replacement	surgical replacement of a coronary valve.
valvotomy	incision into a cardiac valve to remove an obstruction
valvulitis	inflammation of a heart valve.
valvuloplasty	surgical reconstruction of a cardiac valve.
varicose vein	dilated, enlarged, or twisted vein, usually on the leg.
vas(o)	blood vessel
vasoconstrictor	agent that narrows the blood vessels
vasodilator	agent that dilates or widens the blood vessels.
vegetation	clot on a heart valve or opening, usually caused by infection.
vein	any of various blood vessels carrying deoxygenated blood toward the heart, except the pulmonary vein.
vena cava	large vein that transport blood collected from the upper part of the body to the heart. Large vein that draws blood from the lower part of the body to the right atrium.
ven(o)	vein
venipuncture	small puncture into a vein, usually to draw blood or inject a solution.
venography	viewing of a vein by x-ray after injection of a contrast medium.
ventricle	either of the two lower chambers of the heart.
ventriculgram	x-ray of a ventricle taken after injection of a contrast medium.
venule	a tiny vein connecting to a capillary.
AcG	accelerator globulin
AF	atrial fibrillation
AS	aortic stenosis
ASCVD	arteriosclerotic cardiovascular disease
ASD	atrial septal defect
ASHD	arteriosclerotic heart disease
AV	atrioventricular
BP	blood pressure
CABG	coronary artery bypass graft
CAD	coronary artery disease
cath	catheter
CCU	coronary care unit
CHD	coronary heart disease
CHF	congestive heart failure
CO	cardiac output

CPK	creatine phosphokinase
CPR	cardiopulmonary resuscitation
CVA	cerebrovascular accident
CVD	cardiovascular disease
DSA	digital subtraction angiography
DVT	deep venous thrombosis
ECG, EKG	electrocardiogram
ECHO	echocardiogram
ETT	exercise tolerance test
GOT	glutamic oxaloacetic transaminase
HDL	high-density lipoprotein
LDH	lactate dehydroganase
LDL	low-density lipoprotein
LV	left ventricle
LVH	left ventricular hypertrophy
MI	mitral insufficiency; myocardial infarction
MR	mitral regurgitation
MS	mitral stenosis
MUGA	multiple-gated acquisition scan
MVP	mitral valve prolapse
PTCA	percutanceous transluminal coronary angioplasty
PVC	premature ventricular contraction
SA	sinoatrial
SV	stroke volume
tPA, TPA	tissue plasminogen activator
VLDL	very low-density lipoprotein
VSD	ventricular septal defect
VT	ventricular tachycardia
adam's apple	thyroid carilage, supportive structure of the larynx; larger in males than in females.
adenoid(o)	adenoid gland
adenoidectomy	removal of the adenoids
adenoiditis	inflammation of the adenoids.
adenoids	collection of lymphoid tissue in the nasopharynx; pharyngeal tonsils.
alveol(o)	alveolus
alveolus (pl. alveoli)	air sac at the end of each bronchiole.
anthracosis	lung disease caused by long-term in halation of coal dust; black lung disease.
antitussives	agent that control coughing
apex	topmost section of the lung
apnea	cessation of breathing
arterial blood gases	laboratory test that measures the levels of oxygen and carbon dioxide in arterial blood
asbestosis	lung disorder caused by long-term inhalation of asbestos (as in construction work).
asthma	chronic condition with obstruction or narrowing of the bronchial airways.
atelectasis	collapse of a lung or part of a lung.
auscultation	listening to internal sounds with a stethoscope.

bacilli	a type of bacteria
base	bottom section of the lung
black lung	lung disease caused by long-term inhalation of coal dust.
bradypnea	abnormally slow breathing
bronch(o), bronchi(o)	bronchus
bronchial alveolar lavage	retrieval of fluid for examination through a bronchoscope.
bronchial brushing	retrieval of material for biopsy by insertion of a brush through a bronchoscope.
bronchiol(o)	bronchiole
bronchiole	fine subdivision of the bronchi made of smooth muscle and elastic fibers.
bronchitis	inflammation of the bronchi
bronchodilators	agents that dilate the walls of the bronchi
bronchography	radiological picture of the trachea and bronchi
bronchoplasty	surgical repari of a bronchus
bronchoscope	device used to examine airways
bronchospasm	sudden contraction in the bronchi that causes coughing
bronchus (pl. bronchi)	one of the two airways from the trachea to the lungs.
capn(o)	carbon dioxide
Cheyne-Stokes respiration	irregular breathing pattern with a period of apnea followed by deep, labored breathing that becomes shallow, then apneic.
chronic bronchitis	recurring or long-lasting bouts of bronchitis
chronic obstuctive pulmonary disease	disease of the bronchail tubes or lungs with chronic obstruction.
cilia	hairlike extensions of the cell's surface that usually provide some protection by sweeping foreign particles away.
crackles	popping sounds heard in the lung collapse or other conditions; rales
croup	acute respiratory syndrome in children or infants accompanied by seal-like coughing.
cystic fibrosis	disease that causes chronic airway obstruction and also affects the bronchial tubes.
diaphragm	membranous muscle between the abdominal and thoracic cavities that contracts and relaxes during the respiratory cycle.
diphtheria	acute infection of the throat and upper respiratory tract caused by bacteria
dysphonia	hoarseness usually caused by laryngitis
dyspnea	difficult breathing
emphysema	chronic condition of hyperinflation of the air sacs; often caused by prolonged smoking.
empyema	pus in the pleural cavity
endoscope	tube used to view a body cavity
endotracheal intubation	insertion of a tube through the nose or mouth, pharynx, and larynx and into the trachea to establish an airway.
epiglott(o)	epiglottis
epiglottis	cartilaginous flap that covers the larynx during swallowing to prevent food from enerting the airway.
epiglottitis	inflammation of the epiglottis
epistaxis	bleeding from the nose, usually caused by trauma or a sudden rupture of the blood vessels of the nose.
eupnea	normal breathing
exhalation	breathing out
expectorants	agents that promote the coughing and expelling of mucus.

expiration	exhalation
external nares	External openings at the base of the nose; also called external nares
external respiration	exchange of air between the body and the outside enviroment.
glottis	Part of the larynx consisting of the vocal folds of mucous membrane and muscle
Heimlich maneuver	Procedureto prevent choking to death. One person places his or her hands on the midsectionof the choking person's adbomen and thrusts upward until the obstruction is dislodged.
hemoptysis	lung or bronchial hemorrhage resulting in the spitting of blood.
hemothorax	Blood in the pleural cavity
hilum (also hilus)	Midsection of the lung where the nerves and vessels enter and exit.
hypercapnia	Excessive buildup of carbon dioxide in lings, usually associated wht hypoventilation
hyperpnea	Abnormally deep breathing
hyperventilation	Abnormally fast breathing in and out, often associated with anxiety.
hypopharynx	Laryngopharynx
hypopnea	Shallow breathing
hyppoventilation	Abnormally low movement of air in out of the lungs.
hypoxemia	deficient amount of oxygen in the blood.
hypoxia	deficient amount of oxygen in the tissue.
inferior lobe	Bottom lobe of the lung
inhalation	breathing in
inspiration	inhalation
intercostal muscles	muscles between the ribs
internal respiration	exchange of oxygen and carbon dioxide between the cells.
laryng(o)	larynx
laryngectomy	Removal of the larynx
laryngitis	Inflammation of the larynx
laryngocentesis	Surgical puncture of the larynx
laryngopharynx	Part of the pharynx below and behind the larynx
laryngoplasty	Visual examination of the mouth and larynx using an endoscope.
laryngospasm	Sudden contraction of the larynx, which may cause coughing and may restrict breathing.
laryngostomy	Creation of an artificial opening in the larnyx
laryngotracheobronchitis	Inflammation of the larnyx, trachea, and bronchi
laryngotracheotomy	Incision into the larynx and trachea
larynx	Organ of voice production in the respiratory tract, between the pharynx and the trachea; voice box
lob(o)	lobe of the lung
lobeectomy	Removal of one of the lobes of a lung
lung	One of two organs of respiration (left lung and right lung) in the thoracic cavity where oxyegenation of blood takes place
mediastin(o)	mediastinum
mediastinoscopy	Visual examination of the mediastinum and all the organs within it using an endscope
mediastinum	Median portion of the thoracic cavity; septum between two areas of an organ or cavity
mesothelioma	Rare cancer of the lungs assocaited with asbestosis
middle lobe	Middle section of the right lung

nas(O)	nose
nasal cavity	Opening in the external nose where air enters the body
nasal septum	Cartilaginous division of the external nose
nasopharyngitis	Inflammation of the nose and the pharynx
nosopharyngoscopy	Examination of the nasal passages and the pharynx using an endscope
nasopharynx	Portion of the throat above the soft palate
nebulizer	Device that delivers medication through the nose or mouth in a fine spray to the respiratory tract
nose	External structure supported by nasal bones and containing cavity
nosebleed	Bleeding from the nose, usually caused by trauma or a sudden rupture of the blood vessels of the nose.
nostrils	External openings at the base of the nose; also called external nares
or(o)	mouth
oropharynx	Back portion of the mouth, a division of the pharynx
orthopnea	Difficulty in breathing, especially while lying down
otorhinolaryngologist	Medical doctor who diagnoses and treats disorders of the ear, nose and throat
ox(o), oxi, oxy	oxygen
pansinusitis	Inflammation of all the sinuses
paranasal sinuses	Area of the nasal cavity where external air is warmed by blood in the mucous membrane lining
parietal pleura	Outer layer of the pleura
paroxysmal	Sudden, as a spasm or convulsion
peak flow meter	Device for measuring breathing capacity
percussion	Tapping on the surface of the body to see if lungs are clear
pertussis	severe infection of the pharynx, larynx, and trachea caused by bacteria; whooping cough
pharyng(o)	pharynx
pharyngeal tonsils	Adenoids
pharyngitis	Inflammation of the pharynx
pharynx	Passageway at back of mouth for air and food; throat
phon(o)	voice, sound
phren(o)	diaphragm
pleur(o)	pleura
pleura (pl. pleurae)	Double layer of membrane making up the outside of the lungs
pleural cavity	Space between the two pleura
pleural effusion	Escape of fluid into the pleural cavity
pleuritis, pleurisy	Inflammation of the pleura
pleurocentesis	Surgical puncture of pleural space
pleuropexy	Fixing in place of the pleura surgically, usually in case of injury or deterioration
pneum(o), pneumon(o)	air, lung
pneumobronchotomy	incision of the lung and bronchus
pneumoconiosis	Lung condition caused by inhaling dust
pneumonectomy	Removal of a lung
pneumonia	Acute infection of the alveoli
pneumonitis	Inflammation of the lung
pneumothorax	Accumulation of air or gas in the pleural cavity
pulminary abscess	Large collection of pus in the lungs

pulmonary edema	Fluid in the air sacs and brochioles usually caused by failure of the heart to pump enough blood to and from lungs
pulmonary embolism	Clot in the lungs
pulmonary function tests	Tests that measure the mechanics of breathing
rales	Popping sounds heard in lung collapse or other conditions; rales
rhin(o)	nose
rhinitis	Nasal inflammation
rhinoplasty	Surgical repair of the nose
rhinorrhea	Nasal discharge
rhonchi	Whistling sounds heard on inspiration in certain breathing disorders, especially asthma
septoplasty	Surgical repair of the nasal septum
septostomy	Incision of the nasal septum
septum	Cartilaginous division, as in the nose or mediastinum
silicosis	Lung condition caused by silica dust from grinding rocks or glass or other materials used in manufacturing
sungultus	Hiccuping
sinusitis	Inflammation of the sinuses
sinusotomy	Incision of a sinus
soft palate	Flexible muscular sheet that separates the nasopharynx from the rest of the pharynx
spir(o)	breathing
spirometer	Testing maching that measures the lungs' volume and capacity
sputum sample or culture	Cultureof material that is expectorated (or brought back as mucus)
steth(o)	chest
stridor	High-pitched crowing sound heard in certain respiratory conditions
superior lobe	Topmost lobe of each lung
sweat test	Test for cystic fibrosis that measures the amount of salt in sweat.
tachypnea	Abnormally fast breathing
thorac(o)	thorax, chest
thoracic surgeon	Surgeon who specializes in surgery of the thorax
thoracocentesis	Surgical puncture of the chest cavity
thoracostomy	Establishment of an opening in the chest cavity
thoracotomy	Incision into the chest cavity
thorax	Chest cavity
throat	Passageway at back of mouth for air and food; throat
throat culture	Test for streptococcal or other infections in which a swab taken on the surface of the throat is placed in a culture to see if certain bacteria grow
thyroid catilage	Thyroid cartilgae, supportive structure of the larynx; larger in males than in females
tonsil(o)	tonsils
tonsillectomy	Removal of the tonsils
tonsillitis	Inflammation of the tonsils
trachea(o)	trachea
trachea	Airway from the larynx into the bronchi; windpipe
tracheitis	Inflammation of the trachea
tracheoplasty	Repair of the trachea
tracheostomy	Creation of an artificial opening in the trachea

tracheotomy	Incision into the trachea
tuberculosis	Acute infectious disease caused by bacteria called bacilli
upper respiratory infection	Infection of all or part of upper portion of respiratory tract
ventilator	Mechanical breathing device
visceral pleura	Inner layer of the pleura
vocal cords	Strips of epithelial tissue that vibrate and play a major role in the production of sound
voice box	Organ of voice production in the respiratory tract, between the pharynx and the trachea; voice box
wheezes	Whistling sounds heard on inspiration in certain breathing disorders, especially asthma
whooping cough	Severe infection of the pharynx, larynx, and trachea caused by bacteria; whooping cough
windpipe	Airway from the larynx into the bronchi; windpipe
ABG	Arterial blood gases
AFB	Acid-fast bacillus (causes tuberculossis)
A&P	auscultation and percussion
AP	anteroposterior
ARD	adult respiratory disease
ARDS	adult respiratory disease syndrome
ARF	acute respiratory failure
BS	breath sounds
COLD	chronic obstructive lung disease
COPD	chronic obstructive pulmonary disease
CPR	cardiopulmonary resuscitation
CTA	clear to auscultation
CXR	chest x-ray
DOE	dyspnea on exertion
DPT	diphtheria, pertussis, tetanus (combined vaccination)
ENT	ear, nose, and throat
ET Tube	endotracheal intubation tube
FEF	forced expiratory flow
FEV	forced expiratory volume
FVC	forced vital capacity
HBOT	hyperbaric oxygen therapy
IMV	intermittent mandatory ventilation
IPPB	intermittent positive pressure breathing
IRDS	infant respiratory distress syndrome
IRV	inspiratory reserve volume
LLL	left lower lobe (of the lung)
LUL	left upper lobe (of the lung)
MBC	maximal breathing capacity
MDI	metered dose inhaler
PA	posteroanterior
PCP	pneumocystis carininn pneumonia (a type of pneumonia to which AIDS patients are susceptible)
PEEP	postitive and expiratory pressure

PFT	pulmonary function tests
PND	paroxysmal nocturnal dyspnea; postnasal drip
RD	respiratory disease
RDS	respiratory disease syndrome
RLL	right lower lobe (of the lungs)
RUL	right upper lobe (of the lungs)
SIDS	sudden infant death syndrome
SOB	shortness of breath
T&A	tonsillectomy and adenoidectomy
TB	tuberculosis
TLC	total lung capacity
TPR	temperature, pulse, and respiration
URI	upper respiratory infection
VC	vital capacity
V/Q scan	ventilation/perfusion scan
absence seizure	Mild epileptic seizure consisting of brief disorientation with the environment
acetylcholine	Chemical that stimulates cells
afferent neuron	Neuron that carries information from the sensory receptors to the central nervous system
agnosia	Inability to receive and understand outside stimuli
Alzheimer's Disease	Any of variety of degenerative brain diseases causing thought disorders, gradual loss of muscle control, and eventually, death
amnesia	Loss of memory
amyotrophic laterla sclerosis	Degenerative disease of the motor neurons leading to loss muscular control and death
analgesic	Agent that relieves or eliminates pain
anesthetic	Agent that causes loss of feeling or sensation
aneurysm	Abnormal widening of an artery wall that bursts and releases blood
anticonvulsant	Agent that lessens or prevents convulsions
aphasia	Loss of speech
apraxia	Inability to properly use familiar objects
arachnoid	Middle layer of meninges
astrocyte, astroglia	A type of neuroglia that maintains nutrient and chemicals levels in neurons
astrocytoma	Type of glioma formed from astrocytes
ataxia	Condition which uncoordinated voluntary muscular movement, usually resulting from disorders or the cerebellum or spinal cord
aura	Group of sypmtoms that precede a seizure
autonomic nervous system	Part of the peripheral nervous system that carries impulses from the central nervous system to glands, smooth muscles, cardiac muscle, and various membranes
axon	Part of a nerve cell that conducts nerve impulses away from the cell body
bacterial meningitis	Meningitis caused by a bacteria; pyrogenic meningitis
Babinski's reflex	Reflex on the plantar surface of the foot.
basal ganglia	Large masses of gray matter within the cerebrum
Bell's palsy	Paralysis of one side of the face; usually temporary
brain	Body organ responisble for controlling the body's functions and interactions with outside stimuli
brain contusion	Bruising of the surface of the brain without penetration

brainstem	One of the four major divisions of the brain; division that controls certain heart, lung, and visual functions
cell body	Part of a nerve cell that has branches or fibers that reach out to send or receive impulses
central nervous system	Body system consisting of the brain, spinal cord, and meninges
cerebell(o)	cerebellum
cerebellitis	Inflammation of the cerebellum
cerebellum	One of the four major divisions of the brain; division that coordinates musculoskeletal movement
cerebr(o) cerebri	cerebrum
cerebral angiogram	X-ray of the brain's blood vessels after a dye is injected
cerebral cortex	Outer portion of the cerebrum
cerebral infarction	Neurological incident caused by disruption in the normal blood supply to the brain; stroke
cerebral palsy	Congential disease caused by damage to the cerebrum during gestation or birth and resulting in lack of motor coordination.
cerebrospinal fluid	Watery fluid that flows throughout the brain and around the spinal cord
cerebrovascular accident	Neurological incident caused by damage disruption in normal blood supply to the brain;stroke
cerebrum	One of the four major divisions of the brain; division involved with emotions,memory, conscious thought, moral behaviorm sensory interpretations, and certain bodily movement
coma	Abnormally deep sleep with little or no respons to stimuli
computerized (axial) tomography scan	Radiographic imaging that produces cross-sectional images
concussion	Brain injury due to trauma
conductivity	Ability to transmit a signal
convolution	Folds in the cerebral cortex; gyri
cordotomy	Resectioning of a part of the spinal cord
corpus callosum	Bridge of nerve fibers that connects the two hemispheres of the cerebrum
crani(o)	cranium
cranial nerves	Any of 12 pairs of nerves tha tcarry impulses to and from the brain
craniectomy	Removal of a part of the skull
craniotomy	Incision into the skull
dementia	Deterioration in mental capacity, usually in the elderly
demyelination	Destruction of myelin sheath, particularly in MS
dendrite	A thin branching extension of a nerve cell that conducts nerve impulses toward the cell body
diencephalon	One of the four major structures of the brain; it is the deep portion of the brain and contains the thalamus
dopamine	Substance in the brain or manufactured substance that helps relieve symptoms of Parkinson's disease
dura mater	Outermost layer of meninges
duritis	Inflammation of the dura mater
dysphasis	Speech difficulty
efferent neuron	Neuron that carries information to the muscles and glands from the central nervous system
electrencephalogram	Record of the electrical impulses of the brain
embolic stroke	Sudden stroke caused by an embolus
embolus	Clot from somewhere in the body that blocks a small blood vessel in the brain

encephal(o)	brain
encephalitis	Inflammation of the brain
encephalogram	Record of the radiographic study of the ventricles of the brain
epidural space	Area between the pia mater and the bones of the spinal cord
epilepsy	Chronic recurrent seizure activity
epithalamus	One of the parts of the diencephalon; serves as a sensory relay station
evoked potentials	Record of the electrical wave pattern observed in EEG
excitability	Ability to respond to stimuli
fainting	Loss of consciousness due to a sudden lack of oxygen in the brain
fissure	One of may indentations of the cerebrum; sulci
frontal lobe	One of the four parts of each hemisphere of the cerebrum
gait	Manner of walking
gangli(o)	Ganglion
gangliitis	Inflammation of the ganglion
ganglion (pl. ganglia, ganglions)	Any group of nerve cell bodies forming a mass or a cyst in the peripheral nervous system; usually forms in the wrist
gli(o)	neuroglia
glioblastoma multiforme	Most malignant type of glioma
glioma	Tumor that arises from neuroglia
grand mal seizure	Severe epileptic seizure accompanied by convulsions, twitching, and loss of consciouness
gyrus(pl. gyri)	Folds in the cerebral cortex; gyri
hemorrhagic stroke	Stroke caused by blood escaping from a damaged cerebral artery
Huntington's chorea	Hereditary disorder with uncontrollable, jerking movements
hydrocephalus	Overproduction of fluid in the brain
hypnotic	Agent that induces sleep
hypothalamus	One of the parts of the diencephalon; serves as a sensory realy station
interneuron	Neuron that carries and processes sensory information
lobectomy	Removal of a portion of the brain to treat certain disorders
lobotomy	Removal of the frontal lobe of the brain
Lou Gehrig's disease	Degenerative disease of the motor neurons leading to loss of muscular control and death
lumbar puncture	Withdrawal of cerebrospinal fluid from between two lumbar vertebrae
medulla oblongata	Part of the brain stem that regulates hear and lung functions, swallowing, vomiting, coughing, and sneezing
mening(o), meningi(o)	meninges
meninges (sing. meninx)	Three layers of membranes that cover and protect the brain and spinal cord
meningioma	Tumor that arises from the meninges
meningitis	Inflammation of the meninges
meningocele	In spina bifida cystica, protrusion of the spinal meninges above the surface of the skin
meningomyelocele	IN spina bifida cystica, protrusion of the meninges and spinal cord above the surface of the skin
microglia	A type of neuroglia that removes debris
midbrain	Part of the brainstem involved with visual reflexes
multiple sclerosis (MS)	Degenerative disease with loss of myelin, resulting in muscle weakness, extreme fatigue, and some paralysis
myasthenia gravis	Disease involving overproduction of antibodies that block certain

	neurotransmitters; causes muscle weakness
myel(o)	Bone marrow, spinal cord
myelin sheath	Fatty tissue that covers axons
myelitis	Inflammation of the spinal cord
myelogram	X-ray of the spinal cord after a contrast medium has been injected
narcolepsy	Nervous system disorder that causes uncontrollable, sudden lapses into deep sleep
nerve	Bundle of neurons that bear electrical messages to the organs and muscles of the body
nerve cell	Basic cell of the nervous system having three parts: cell body, dendrite, and axon; neuron
nerve conduction velocity	Timing of the conductivity of an electrical shock administered to peripheral nerves
nerve impulse	Release energy that is received or transmitted by tissue or organs and that usually provokes a response
neur(o), neuri	nerve
neurectomy	Surgical removal of a nerve
narcotic	Agent that relieves pain by inducing a stuporous or euphoric state
neurilemma	Membranous covering that protects the myelin sheath
neuritis	Inflammation of the nerves
neuroglia, neuroglial	Cell of the nervous system that does not transmit impulse
neuron	Basic cell of the nervous systen having three parts; nerve cell
neuroplasty	Surgical repair of a nerve
neurorrhaphy	Suturing of a severed nerve
neurosurgeon	Medical specialist who performs surgery on the brain and spinal cord
neurotomy	Dissection of a nerve
neurotransmitter	various substances located in tiny sacs at the end of the axon
occipital lobe	One of the four parts of each hemisphere of the cerebrum
occlusion	Blocking of a blood vessel
oligodendroglia	A type of neuroglia that produces myelin and helps support neurons
oligodendroglioma	Type of glioma formed from oligodendroglia
palsy	Partial or complete paralysis
parasympathetic nervous system	Part of the autonomic nervous system that operates when the body is in a normal state
parietal lobe	One of the four part of each hemisphere of the cerebrum
Parkinson's disease	Degeneration of nerves in the brain caused by lack of sufficient dopmanine
PET (positron emission tomography)	Imaging of the brain using radioactive isotopes and tomography
petit mal seizure	Mild epileptic seizure consisting of brief cisorientation with the environment
pia mater	Innermost layer of meninges
polysomnography	Recording of electrical and movement patterns during sleep
pons	Part of the brainstem that controls certain respiratory functions
pyrogenic meningitis	Meningitis caused by bacteria; can be fatal; bacterail meningitis
radiculitis	Inflammation of the spinal nerve roots
receptor	Tissue or organ that receives nerve impulses
reflex	Involuntary muscular contraction in response to a stimulus
sciatica	Inflammation of the sciatic nerve
sedative	Agent that relieves feeling of agitation

shingles	Viral disease affecting the peripheal nerves
somatic nervous system	Part of the peripheral nervous system that receives and processes sensor input from various parts of the body
somnambulsim	Sleepwalking
somnolence	Extreme sleepiness caused by a neurological disorder
SPECT (single photon emission computed tomography) brain scan	Brain image produced by the use of radioactive isotopes
spin(o)	spine
spina bifida	Congential defect of the spinal column
spinal cord	Ropelike tissue that sits inside the vertebral column and from which spinal nerves extend
spinal nerves	Any of 31 pairs of nerves that carry messages to and from the spinal corn and the torso and extremities
sterotaxy or stereotactic surgery	Destruction of deep-seated brain structures using three-dimensional coordinates to locate the structures
stimulus (pl. stimuli)	Anything that arouses a response
stroke	Neurological incident caused by disruption in the normal blood supply to the brain; stroke
subdural space	Area between the dura mater and pia mater across which the arachnoid runs
sulcus (pl.sulci)	One of many indentations of the cerebrum; sulci
sympathetic nervous system	Of the part of the autonomic nervous system that operates when the body is under stress
synapse	Space over which nerve impulses jump from one neuron to another
syncope	Loss of consciousness due to a sudden lack of oxygen to the brain
Tay-Sachs disease	Hereditary disease that causes deterioration in the central nervous system and eventually, death
temporal lobe	One of the four parts of each hemisphere of the cerebrum
terminal end fibers	Group of fibers at the end of an axon that passes the impulses leaving the neuron to the next neuron
thalam(o)	thalamus
thalamus	One of the four parts of the diencephalon; serves as a sensory relay station
thrombotic stroke	Stroke caused by a thrombus
thrombus	Blood clot
tics	Twitching movement that accompany some neurological disorders
tonic-clonic seizure	Severe epileptic seizure accompanied by convulsions, twitching, and loss of consciousness
trancranial sonogram	Brain images produced by the use of sound waves
trephination	Circular incision into the skull
Tourette syndrome	Neurological disorders that causes uncontrollable speech sounds and tics
transient ischemic attack	Short neurological incident usually not resulting in permanent injury, but usually signaling that a larger stroke may occur
vag(o)	vagus nerve
vagotomy	Surgical cutting off of the vagus nerve
ventral thalamus	One of the four parts of the diencephalon; serves as a sensory relay station
ventricle	Cavity in the brain for cerebrospinal fluid
ventricul(o)	ventricle
viral meningitis	Meningitis caused by a virus and not as severe as pyrogenic meningitis
Ach	acetylcholine

ALS	amyotrophic lateral sclerosis
BBB	blood-brain barrier
CNS	central nervous system
CP	cerebral palsy
CSF	cerebrospinal fluid
CT or CAT scan	computerized (axial) tomography
CVA	cerebrovascular accident
CVD	cerebrovascular disease
EEG	electroencephalogram
ICP	intracranial pressure
LP	lumbar puncture
MRA	magnetic resonance angiography
MRI	magnetic resonance imaging
SAH	subarachnoid hemorrhage
TIA	transient ischemic attack
acetone	Type of ketone normally found in urine in small quantities; found in larger quantities in diabetic urine
albumin	Simple protein; when leaked into urine, may indicate a kidney problem
albuminuria	Presence of albumin in urine, usually indicative of disease
antispamodic	Pharmacological agent that relieves spasms; also decreases frequency of urination
anuresis	Abnormal retention of urine
anuria	Lack of urine formation
atresia	Abnormal narrowing, as of the ureters or urethra
azotemia	Excess of urea and other wastes in the blood
bilirubin	Substance produced in the liver; elevated levels may indicate liver disease or hepatitis when found in urine
bladder	Organ where urine collects before being excreted from the body
bladder cancer	Malignancy of the bladder
Bowman's capsule	Capsule surrounding a glomerulus and serving as a collection site for urine
Bright's disease	Inflammation of the glomeruli that can result in kidney failure
cali(o), calic(o)	calix
calices, calyces, (sing. calix, calyx)	Cup-shaped structures in the renal pelvis for the collection of urine
casts	materials formed in urine when protein accumlates; may indicate renal disease
condom catheter	Disposable catheter for urinary sample collection or incontinence
cortex	Outer portion of the kidney
creatine	Substance found in urine; elevated levels may indicate muscular dystrophy
creatinine	A component creatine
cyst(o)	bladder
cystectomy	Surgical removal of the bladder
cystitis	Inflammation of the bladder
cystocele	Hernia of the bladder
cystolith	Bladder stone
cystopexy	Surgical fixing of the bladder to the abdominal wall
cystoplasty	Surgical repair of the bladder
cystorrhaphy	Suturing of a damaged bladder

cystoscope	Tubular instrument for examining the interior of the bladder
cystoscopy	Tubular instrument for examining the inerior of the bladder
dialysis	Method of filtration used when kidneys fail
diuretic	Pharmacological agent that increases urination
dysuria	Painful urination
edema	Retention of water in cells, tissues, and cavities, sometimes due to kidney disease
end-stage-renal disease (ESRD)	The last stage of kidney failure
enuresis	Urinary incontinence
extracorporeal shock wave lithotripsy (ESWL)	Breaking of kidney stones by using shock waves from outside the body
filtration	Process of separating solids from a liquid by passing it through a porous substance
Foley catheter	Indwelling catheter held in place by a balloon that inflates inside the bladder
glomerul(o)	glomerulus
glomerulonephritis	Inflammation of the glomeruli of the kidneys
glomerulus (pl. glomuleri)	Group of capillaries in a nephron
glucose	Form of sugar found in the blood; may indicate diabetes when found in the urine
hematuria	Blood in the urine
hemodialysis	Dialysis performed by passing blood through a filter outside the body and returning filtered blood to the body
hilum	Portion of the kidney where blood vessels and nerves enter and exit
hydronephrosis	Abnormal collection of urine in the kidneys due to a blockage
incontinence	Inability to prevent excretion of urine or feces
indwelling	Of a type of catheter inserted into a body
intracorporeal electrohydraulic lithotripsy	Use of an endoscope to break up stones
ketone	Substance that reults from the breakdown of fat; indicates diabetes of starvation when present in the urine
ketonuria	Increased urinary excretion of ketones, usually indicative of diabetes or starvation
kidney	Organ tha forms urine and reaborbs essentail substances back into the bloodstream
kidney failure	Loss of kidney function
kidney, ureter, bladder (KUB)	X-ray of three parts of the urinary system
lithotomy	Surgical removal of bladder stones
meato	meatus
meatotomy	Surgical enlargement of the meatus
meatus	External opening of a canal, such as the urethra
medulla	Soft, central portion of the kidney
nephrectomy	Removal of a kidney
nephritis	Inflammation of the kidneys
nephro(o)	kidney
nephroblastoma	Malignant kidney tumor found primarily in young children; nephroblastoma
nephrolithotomy	Surgical removal of a kidney stone

nephrolysis	Removal of kidney adhersions
nephroma	Any renal tumor
nephron	Functional unit of a kidney
nephropexy	Surgical fixing of a kidney to the abdominal wall
nephrorrhaphy	Suturing of a damaged kidney
nephrosis	Disorder caused by loss of protein in the urine
nephrostomy	Establsihment of an opening from the renal pelvis to the outside of the body
nocturia	Nighttime urination
oliguria	Scanty urine production
peritoneal dialysis	Type of dialysis in which liquid that extracts substances from blood is inserted into the peritoneal cavity and emptied outside the body
pH	Measurement of the acidity or alkalinity of a solution such as urine
phenylketones	Substances that, if accumulated in the urine of infants, indicate phenylketonuria, a disease treated by diet
polycystic kidney disease	Condition with many cysts on and within the kidneys
polyuria	Excessive urination
prostate	Gland surrounding the urethra in the male; active in ejaculation of semen
proteinuria	Abnormal presence of protein in the urine
pyel(o)	renal pelvis
pyelitis	Inflammation of the renal pelvis
pyeloplasty	Surgical repair of the renal pelvis
pyelotomy	Incision into the renal pelvis
pyuria	Pus in the urine
reabsorption	Process of returning essential elements to the bloodstream after filtration
ren(o)	Kidney
renal pelvis	Collectin area for urine in the center of the kidney
renin	Enzyme produced in the kidneys to regulate the filtration rate of blood by increasing blood pressure as necessary
renogram	Radioactive imaging of kidney function after introduction of a substance that is filtered through the kidney while it is observed
resectoscope	type of endoscope for removal of lesions
retrograde pyelogram	X-ray of the bladder and ureters after a contrast medium is injected into the bladder
retroperitoneal	Posterior to the peritoneum
specific gravity	Measurement of the concentration of wastes, minerals, and solids in urine
trigon(o)	trigone
trigone	Triangular area at the base of the bladder through which the ureters enter and the urethra exits the bladder
ur(o) urin(o)	urine
urea	waste product of nitrogen metabolism excreted in normal adult urine
uremia	Excess of urea and other wastes in the blood
ureter(o)	ureter
ureterctomy	Surgical removal of all or some of a ureter
ureteroplasty	Surgical repair of a ureter
ureterorrhaphy	Suturing of a ureter
urethr(o)	urethra
urethra	Tube through which urine is transported from the bladder ti the exterior of the body

urethropexy	Surgical fixing of the urethra
urethroplasty	Surgical repair of the urethra
urethrorrhaphy	Suturing of the urethra
urethrostomy	Establishment of an opening between the urethra and the exterior of the body
urethrotomy	Surgical incision of a narrowing in the urethra
uric acid	Nitrogenous waste excreted in the urine
urinalysis	Examination of the properties of urine
urinary bladder	Organ where urine collects before being excreted from the body
urinary system	body system that forms and excretes urine and helps in the reabsorption of essential substances
urinary tract infection	Infection of the urinary tract
urine	Fluid excreted by the urinary system
urology	Medical specialty that diagnoses and treats the urinary system and the male reproductive system
urostomy	Establishment of am opening in the abdomen to the exterior of the body for the release of urine
vesic(o)	bladder
voiding (urinating) cystourethogram (VCU, VCUG)	X-ray image made after indroduction of a contrast medium and while urination is taking place
Wilms' Tumor	Malignant kidney tumor found primarily in young children; nephroblastoma
ADH	antidiuretic hormone
A/G	albumin/globulin
AGN	acute glomerulonephritis
ARF	acute renal failure
ATN	acute tubular necrosis
BNO	bladder neck obstruction
BUN	blood urea nitrogen
CAPD	continuous ambulatory peritoneal dialysis
Cath	catheter
Cl	chlorine
CRF	chronic renal failure
cysto	cystoscopy
ESRD	end-stage renal disease
ESWL	extracorporeal shock wave lithotripsy
HD	hemodialysis
IVP	intravenous pyelogram
K+	potassium
KUB	kidney, ureter, bladder
Na+	sodium
pH	power of hydrogen concentration
PKU	phenylketonuria
RP	retrograde pyelogram
SG	specific gravity
UA	urinalysis
UTI	urinary tract infection
VCU, VCUG	voiding cystourethrogram
abortion	Premature ending of a pregnancy

abortifacient	Medication to prevent implantation of an ovum
abruptio placnetae	Breaking away of the placenta from the uterine wall
afterbirth	Placenta and membranes that are expelled from the uterus afterbirth
amenoorrhea	Lack of menstruation
amni(o)	amnion
amniocentesis	Removal of a sample of amniotic fluid through a needle injected in the amniotic sac
anovulation	Lack of ovulation
anteflexion	Bending forward, as of the uterus
areola	Darkish area surrounding the nipple on a breast
aspiration	Biopsy in which fluid is withdrawn through a needle by suction
Bartholin's gland	One of two glands on either side of the vagina that secrete fluid into the vagina
birth control pills or implants	Medication that controls the flow of hormones to block ovulation
body	Middle portion of the uterus
carcinoma in situ	Localized malignancy that has not spread
cauterization	Removal or destruction of tissue using chemicals or devices, such as laser-guided equipment
cervic(o)	cervix
cervicitis	Inflammation of the cervix
cervix	Protective part of uterus, located at the bottom and protruding through the vaginal wall; contains glands that secrete fluid into the vagina
chlamydia	Sexually transmitted bacterial infection affecting various parts of the male or female reproductive systems; the bacterial agent itself
chorion	Outermost membrane of the sac surrounding the fetus during gestation
climacteric	Period of hormonal changes just prior to menopause
clitoris	Primary organ of female sexual stimulation, located at the top of the labia minora
coitus	Sexual intercourse
colp(o)	vagina
colposcopy	Examination of the vagina with colposcope
condom	Contraceptive device consisting of a rubber or vinyl sheath placed over the penis or as lining that covers the vaginal canal that blocks contact between the sperm and the female sex organs
condyloma	Growth on the external genitalia
conization	Removal of a cone-shaped section of the cervix for examination
contraception	Method of controlling conception by blocking access or interrupting reproductive cycles; birth control
copulation	Sexual intercourse
corpus luteum	Structure formed after the graafian follicle fills with a yellow substance that secretes estrogen and progesterone
cryosurgery	Removal or destruction of tissue using cold temperatures
culdocentesis	Taking of a fluid sample from the base of the pelvic cavity to see if an ectopic pregnancy has ruptured
culdoscopy	Examination of the pelvic cavity using an endoscope
diaphragm	Contraceptive device that covers the cervix and blocks sperm from entering; used in conjunction with spermicide
dysmenorrhea	Painful menstruation
dyspareunia	Painful sexaul intercourse due to any of various conditions, such as cysts,

	infection, or dryness, in the vagina
endometriosis	Abnormal condition in which uterine wall tissue is found in the pelvis or on the abdominal wall
endometrium	Inner mucous layer of the uterus
episi(o)	vulva
estrogen	One of the primary female hormones produced by the ovaries
fallopian tube	One of two tubes that lead from the ovaries to the uterus; uterine tube
fibroid	Benign tumor commonly found in the uterus
fimbriae	Hairlike ends of the uterine tubes that sweep the ovum into the uterus
follicle-stimulating hormone (FSH)	Hormone necessary for maturation of oocytes and ovulation
foreskin	Fold of skin at the top of the labia minora
fundus	Top portion of the uterus
galact(o)	milk
gamete	Sex cell; mature female sex cell produced by teh ovaries, which then travels to the uterus. If fertilized, it implants in the uterus; if not, it is released during menstruation to the outside of the body
gestation	Period of fetal development in the uterus; usually about 40 weeks
gonad	Male or female sex organ; one of two glands that produce ova
gonorrhea	Sexually transmitted inflammation of the genital membranes
graafian follicle	Follicle in the ovary that holds an oocyte during development and then releases it.
gravida	Pregnant woman
gynec(o)	Female
gynecologist	Specialist who diagnoses and treats the processes and disorders of the female reproductive system
hormone	Chemical secretion from glands such as the ovaries
hormone replacement therapy (HRT)	Treatment with hormones when the body stops or decreases the production of hormones by itself
hymen	Fold of mucous membranes covering the vagina of a young female; usually ruptures during first intercourse
hyster(o)	uterus
hysteroctomy	Removal of the uterus
hysterosalpingography	X-ray of the uterus and uterine tubes after a contrast medium has been injected
hysteroscopy	Examination of the uterus using a hysteroscope
intrauterine device (IUD)	Contraeceptive device consisting of a coil placed in the uterus to block implantation of a fertilized ovum
introitus	External openings or entrance to a hollow organ, such as a vagina
isthmus	Narrow region at the bottom of the uterus opening into the cervix
Kegal exercises	Exercise to strengthen pubic muscles
labia majora	Two folds of skin that form the borders of the vulva
labia minora	Two folds of skin between the labia majora
lact(o), lacti	milk
lactation	Production of milk from the breasts following delivery
lactiferous	Producing milk
laparoscopy	Use of a lighted tubular instrument inserted through a woman's naval to perform a tubal ligation or to examine the fallopian tubes
leukorrhea	Abnormal vaginal discharge; usually whitish
lumpectomy	Removal of a breast tumor

luteinizing hormone (LH)	Hormone essential ot ovulation
mamm(o)	breast
mammary glands	Glandular tissue that forms the breasts, which respond to cycles of menstuation and birth
mammography	X-ray imaging of the breast as a cancer screening method
mammoplasty	Plastic surgery to reconstruct the breast, particularly after a mastectomy
mast(o)	breast
mastectomy	Removal of a breast
mastitis	Inflammation of the breast
mastopexy	Surgical procedure to attach sagging breasts in a more normal postion
men(o)	menstruation
menarche	First menstruation
menometrorrhagia	Irregular or excessive bleeding between or during menstruation
menopause	Time when menstruation ceases; usually between ages 45 and 55
menorrhagia	Excessive menstrual bleeding
menstruation	Cyclical release of uterine lining through the vagina; usually every 28 days
metr(o)	uterus
metrorrhagia	Uterine bleeding between menstrual periods
miscarriage	Spontaneous, premature ending of a pregnancy
mons pubis	Mound of soft tissue in the external genitalia covered by pubic hair after puberty
morning-after pill	Medication to prevent implantation of an ovum
myomectomy	Removal of fibroids from the uterus
myonmetrium	Middle layer of muscle tissue of the uterus
nipple	Projection of the apex of the breast through which milk flows during lactation
oo	egg
obstetrician	Physician who specializes in pregnancy and childbirth care
oligomenorrhea	Scanty menstrual period
oligo-ovulation	Irregular ovulation
oocyte	Immature ovum produced in the gonads
oophor(o)	ovary
oophorectomy	Removal of an ovary
ov(i), ov(o)	egg
ovari(o)	ovary
ovulation	Release of an ovum(or rarely, more than one ovum) as part of monthly cycle that leads to fertilization or menstruation
ovum (pl. ova)	Mature female sex cell produced by the ovaries, which then travels to the uterus. If fertilized, it implants in the uterus; if not, it is released during menstruation to the outside of the body
oxytocin	Hormone given to induce labor
Papanicolaou smear	Gathering of cells from the cervix and vagina to observe for abnormalities
para	Woman who has given birth to one or more viable infants
parturition	Birth
pelvimetry	Measurement of the pelvis during pregnancy
perimenopause	Three-to-five-year period of decreasing estrogen levels prior to menopause
perimetrium	Outer layer of the uterus
perine(o)	perineum
perineum	Space between the labia majora and the anus

placenta	Nutrient-rich organ that develops in the uterus during pregnancy; supplies nutrients to the fetus
placenta previa	Placement of the placenta so it blocks the birth canal
preclampsia	Toxic infection during pregnancy
progesterone	One of the primary female hormones
puberty	Pre-teen or early teen period when secondary sex characteristics develop and menstruation begins
retroflexion	Bending backward of the uterus
retroversion	Backward turn of the uterus
salping(o)	fallopian tube
salpingectomy	Removal of a fallopian tube
salpingitis	Inflammation of the fallopian tube
salpingotomy	Incision into the fallopian tube
sinus	Space between the lactiferous ducts and the nipple
spermicide	Contraceptive chemical that destroys sperm; usually in cream or jelly form
sponge	Polyurethane contraceptive device filled with spermicide and placed in vagina near cervix
syphilis	Sexually transmitted acute infection
tocolytic agent	Hormone given to stop labor
umbilical cord	Cord that connects the placenta in the mother's uterus to the navel of the fetus during gestation for nourishment of the fetus
uter(o)	uterus
uterine tube	One of two tubes through which ova travel from an ovary to the uterus
uterus	Female reproductive organ; site of implantation after fertilization or release of the lining during menstruation
vagin(o)	vagina
vaginitis	Inflammation of the vagina
vulv(o)	vulva
vulva	External female genitalia
AB	abortion
AFP	alpha fetoprotein
AH	abdominal hysterectomy
CIS	caricinoma in situ
CS	caesarean section
C-section	caesarean section
Cx	cervix
D&C	dilation and curettage
DES	diethylsilbestrol
DUB	dysfunctional uterine bleeding
ECC	endocervical curettage
EDC	expected date of confinement
EMB	endometrial biopsy
ERT	estrogen replacement therapy
FHT	fetal heart tones
FSH	follicle-stimulating hormone
G	gravida (pregnancy)
gyn	gynecology

HCG	human chorionic gonadotropin
HRT	hormone replacement therapy
HSG	hysterosalpingography
HSO	hysterosalpingoophorectomy
IUD	intrauterine device
LH	luteinizing hormone
LMP	last menstrual period
multip	multiparous
OB	obstetrics
OCP	oral contraceptive pill
P	para (live birth)
Pap smear	Papanicolaou smear
PID	pelvic inflammatory disease
PMP	previous menstrual period
PMS	premenstrual syndrome
primip	primiparous
TAH-BSO	total abdominal hysterectomy with bilateral salping oophorectomy
TSS	toxic shock syndrome
UC	uterine contractions
anabolic steriods	Prescription drug abused by some athletes to increase muscle mass
andr(o)	men
anorchism, anorchia	Congenital absence of one or both testicles
aspermia	Inability to produce sperm
azoospermia	Semen without living sperm
balan(o)	glans penis
balanitis	Inflammation of the glans penis
bulbourethral gland	One of two glands below the prostate that secrete a fluid to lubricate the inside of the urethra
castration	Removal of the testicles
chancroids	Bacterial infection that can be sexually transmitted; results in sores on the penis, urethra, or anus
circumcision	Removal of the foreskin
Cowper's gland	One of two glands below the prostate that secretes a fluid to lubricate the inside of the urethra
cryptorchism	Birth defect with the failure of one or both of the testicles to descend in to the scrotal sac
ejaculation	Expulsion of semen outside the body
epididym(o)	epididymis
epididymectomy	Removal of an epididymis
epididymis	Group of ducts at the top of the testis where sperm are stored
epididymitis	Inflammation of the epididymis
epispadias	Birth defect with abnormal opening of the urethra on the top side of the penis
flagellum	Tail at the end of a sperm that helps it move.
foreskin	Flap of skin covering the glans penis; removed by circumcision in many cultures
glans penis	Sensitive area at the tip of the penis
hernia	Abnormal protrusion of tissue through muscle that contains it
hydrocele	Fluid-containing hernia of the testis

hypospadias	Birth defect with abnormal opening of the urethra on the bottom side of the penis
impotence	Inability to maintain an erection for ejaculation
infertility	Inability to fertilize ova
oligospermia	Scanty production of sperm
orch(o), orchi(o), orchid(o)	testes
orchidectomy	Removal of a testicle
orchiectomy	Removal of a testicle
penis	Male reproductive part that covers the urethra on the outside of the body
perineum	Area between the penis and the anus
Peyronie's disease	Abnormal curvature of the penis caused by hardening in the interior of the penis
phimosis	Abnormal narrowing of the opening of the foreskin
prostat(o)	prostate gland
prostate gland	Gland surrounding the urethra that emits fluid to help sperm move and contracts its muscular tissue during ejaculation to help the sperm exit the body
prostatectomy	Removal of the prostate
prostate-specific antigen test	Blood test for prostate cancer
prostatitis	Inflammation of the prostate
scrotum	Sac outside the body containing the testicles
semen	Thick, whitish fluid containing spermatozoa and secretions from the seminal vesicles, Cowper's glands, and prostate; ejaculated from the penis
semen analysis	Observation of semen for viability of sperm
seminoma	Malignant tumor of the testicles
sperm	Male sex cell that contains chromosomes
sperm(o) spermat(o)	sperm
spermatozoon (pl. spermatozoa)	Male sex cell that contains chromosomes
testicles	Male organ that produces sperm and is contained in the scrotum
testis (pl. testes)	Male organ that produces sperm and is contained in the scrotum
testosterone	Primary male hormone
urethrogram	X-ray of the urethra and prostate
varicocele	Enlargement of veins of the spermatic cord
vas deferens	Narrow tube through which sperm leave the epididymis and travel to the seminal vesicles and into the urethra
vasectomy	Removal of part of the vas deferens to prevent conception
vasovasostomy	Reversal of a vasectomy
AIH	artificial insemination homogous
BPH	benign prostatic hypertrophy
PED	penile erectile dysfunction
PSA	prostate-specific antigen
SPP	suprapibic prostatectomy
TURP	transurethral resection of the prostate
agglutin(o)	agglutinin
agglutination	Clumping of cells and particles in blood
agglutinogen	Substance that causes agglutination

agranulocyte	Leukocyte with nongranular cytoplasm
albumin	Simple protein found in plasma
anemia	Condition in which red blood cells do not transport enough oxygen to the tissues
anisocytosis	Condition with abnormal variation in the size of red blood cells
anticoagulant	Agent that prevents formation of blood clots
antiglobulin test	Test for antibodies on red blood cells
basophil	Leukocyte containing heparin and histamine and performing a phagocytic function
basophilia	Condition with an increased number of basophils in the blood
biochemistry panel	Common group of automated tests run on one blood sample
blood	Fluid (containing plasma, red blood cells, white blood cells, and platelets) circulated throughout the arteries, veins, capillaries, and heart
blood chemistry	Test of plasma for presence of a particular substance such as glucose
blood culture	Test of a blood specimen in a culture medium to observe for particular mocroorganisms
blood indices	Measurement of the characteristics of red blood cells
blood types or groups	Classification of blood according to its antigen and anitbody qualities
bone marrow biopsy	Extraction of bone marrow, by means of a needle for observation
bone marrow transplant	Injection of donor bone marrow into a patient whose diseased cells have been killed through radiation and chemotherapy
chemistry profile	test of plasma for presence of a particular substance such as glucose
coagulant	Clotting agent
coagulation	Changing of a liquid, especially blood, into a semi-solid
complete blood count (CBC)	Most common blood test for a number of factors
dyscrasia	Any disease with abnormal particles in the blood
electrophoresis	Process of separating particles in a solution by passing electricity through the liquid
eosino	eosinophil
eosinophil	Type of granulocyte
eosinophilia	Condition with an abnormal number of eosinophils in the blood
erythr(o)	red
erythroblastosis fetalis	Incompatibility disoreder between a mother with Rh negative and a fetus with Rh positive
erythrocyte	Mature red blood cell
erythrocyte sedimentation rate (ESR)	Test for rate at which red blood cells fall through plasma
erythropenia	Disorder with abnormally low number of red blood cells
erythropoietin	Hormone released by the kidneys to stimulate red blood cell production
fibrin clot	Clot-forming threads formed at the site of an injury during coagulation where platelets clump together with various other substances
fibrinogen	Protein in plasma that aids in clotting
gamma globulin	Globulin that arises in lymphatic tissue and functions as part of the immune system
globin	Protein molecule; in blood, a part of hemoglobin
granulocyte	Leukocyte with granular cytoplasm
granulocytosis	Condition with abnormal number of granulocytes in the bloodstream
hematocrit	Measure of the percentage of red blood cells in a blood sample

hematocytoblast	Most immature blood cell
heme	Pigment containing iron in hemoglobin
hemo hemat(o)	blood
hemochromatosis	Hereditary condition with excessive iron buildup in the blood
hemoglobin	Protein in red blood cells essential to the transport of oxygen
hemolsis	Disorder with breakdown of red blood cell membranes
hemophilia	Hereditary disorder with lack of clotting factor in the blood
hemostatic	Agent that stops bleeding
heparin	Substance in blood that prevents clotting
histamine	Substance released by basophils and eosinophils; involved in allergic reations
leuk(o)	white
leukocyte	Mature white blood cell
lymphocyte	Type of agranulocyte
macrocytosis	Disorder with abnormally large red blood cells
megakaryocyte	Large cells in red bone barrow that form platelets
microcytosis	Disorder with abnormally small red blood cells
monocyte	Type of agranulocyte
multiple myeloma	Malignant tumor of the bone marrow
myeloblast	Immature granulocytes
neurtrophil	Type of leukocyte; granulocyte
pancytopenia	Condition with low number of blood components
partial thromboplastin time (PTT)	Test for ability of blood to coagulate
phag(o)	eating, devouring
phlebotomy	Insertion of a needle into a vein, usually for the purpose of extracting a blood sample
plasma	Liquid portion of unclotted blood
plasmapheresis	Process of removing blood from a person, centrifuging it, and returning only red blood cells to that person
platelet	Thrombocyte; part of a megakaryocyte that initiates clotting
platelet count (PLT)	Measurement of number of platelets in a blood samples
poikilocytosis	Disorder with irregularly shaped red blood cells
polycythemia	Disorder with abnormal increase in red blood cells and hemoglobin
prothrombin time (PT)	Test ability of blood to coagulate
purpura	Condition with multiple, tiny hemorrhages under the skin
red blood cell	One of the solid parts of blood formed from stem cells and having hemoglobin within; erythrocyte
red blood cell count	Measurement of red blood cells in a cubic millimeter of blood
red blood cell morphology	Observation of shape of red blood cells
relapse	Recurrence of a disease
remission	Disappearance of a disease for a time
reticulocytosis	Disorder with an abnormal number of immature erthrocytes
Rh factor	Type of antigen in blood that can cause a transfusion reaction
Rh-negative	Lacking Rh factor on surface of blood cells
Rh-positive	Having Rh factor on surface on blood cells
sedimentation rate (SR)	Test for rate at which red blood cells fall through plasma
serum	The liquid left after blood had clotted

SMA (sequential multiple analyzer)	Original blood chemistry machine; now a synonym for blood chemistry
stem cell	Immature cell formed in bone marrow that becomes differentiated into either a red or a white blood cell
thalassemia	Hereditary disorder characterized by inability to produce sufficient hemoglobin
thromb(o)	blood clot
thrombin	Enzyme that helps in clot formation
thrombocyte	Platelet; cell fragment that produces thrombin
thrombocytopenia	Bleeding condition with insufficient production of platelets
thrombolytic	Agent that disolves blood clots
thromboplastin	Protein that aids in forming a fibrin clot
transfusion	Injection of donor blood into a person needing blood
venipucture	Insertion of a needle into a vein, usually for the purpose of extracting a blood sample
von Willebrand's disease	Hemorrhagic disorder with tendency to bleed from mucous membranes
white blood cell	One of the solid parts of blood from stem cells that plays a role in defense against disease; leukocyte
APTT	activated partial thromboplastin time
baso	basophil
BCP	biochemistry panel
BMT	bone marrow transplant
CBC	complete blood count
diff	differential blood count
eos	eosinophils
ESR	erythrocyte sedimentation rate
G-CSF	Granulocyte colony-stimulating factor
GM-CSF	Granulocyte macrophage colony stimulating factor
HCT, Hct	hematocrit
HGB, Hgb, HB	hemoglobin
MCH	mean corpuscular hemoglobin
MCHC	mean corpuscular hemoglobin concentration
MCV	mean corpuscular volume
mono	monocyte
PCV	packed cell volume
PLT	platelet count
PMN, poly	polymorphonuclear neurtrophil
PT	prothrombin time
PTT	partial thromboplastin time
RBC	red blood cell count
SR; sed,rate	sedimentation rate
seg	segmented mature white blood cells
WBC	white blood cell count
acquired active immunity	Resistance to a disease acquired naturally or developed by previous exposure or vaccination
acquired passive immunity	Inoculation against disease or poison, using antitoxins or antibodies from or in another person or another species
acquired immunodeficiency	AIDS

	disease
aden(o)	gland
allergen	Substance to which exposure causes an allergic reaction
allergy	Production of IgE antibodies against an allergen
anaphylaxis	Life-threatening allergic reaction
anntibody	Specialized protein that fights disease
antigen	any substance in the bloodstream that can provoke an immune response
antitoxin	Antibodies directed against a particular disease or poison
autoimmune disease	Any of a number of diseases, such as rheumatoid arthritis, lupus, and scleroderma, caused by an autoimmune response
autoimmune response	Overactivity in the immune system against oneself causing destruction of one's own healthy cells
cell-mediated immunity	Resistance to disease mediated by T cells
cytotoxic cell	T cell that helps in destruction of infected cells throught out the body
enzyme-linked immunosorbent assay (EIA, ELISA)	Test used to screen blood for the presence of antibodies to different viruses or bacteria
gamma globulin	Antibodies given to prevent or lessen certain diseases
helper cell	t cell that stimulates the immune response
histiocytic lymphoma	Lymphoma with malignant cells that resemble histiocytes
Hodgkin's lymphoma, Hodgkin's disease	Type of lymph cancer of uncertain origin that generally appears in early adulthood
human immunodeficiency virus (HIV)	Virus that causes AIDS; spread by sexual contact and exchange of body fluids
humoral immunity	Resistance to disease provided by plasma cells and anitbody production
hypersensitivity	Abnormal reaction to an allergen
hypersplenism	Overactive spleen
immun(o)	immunity
immunity	Resistance to particular pathogens
immunoglobulin	Type of antibody
immunosuppressive disease	Disease that flourishes because of lowered immune response
infectious mononucleosis	Acute infectious disease caused by the Epstein-Barr virus
interferon	Protein produced by T cells and other cells; destroys disease-causing cells with its antiviral properties
interleukin	Protein produced by T cells; helps regulates immune system
lymph	Fluid containing white blood cells and toher substances that flows in the lymphactic vessels
lymph(o)	lymph
lymphaden(o)	lymph nodes
lymphadenectomy	Removal of a lymph node
lymphadenopathy	Swollen lymph nodes
lymphadenotomy	Incision into a lymph nodes
lymphangi(o)	lymphatic vessels
lymph node	Specialized organ that produces lymphocytes and filters harmful substances from the tissues
lymph node dissection	Removal of a cancerous node for microscopic examination
lymphocytes	Lymph cells

lymphocytic lymphoma	Lymphoma with malignant cells that resemble large lymphocytes
lymphoma	Cancer of the lymph nodes
macrophage	Special cell that devours foreign substances
metastasis	Spread of a cancer from a localized area
natural immunity	Inherent resistance to disease found in a species, race, family group, or certain individuals
non-Hodgkin's lymphoma	Cancer of the lymph nodes with some cells resembling healthy cells and spreading in a diffuse pattern
opportunistic infection	Infection that takes hold because of lowered immune response
pathogen	Disease-causing agent
phagocytosis	Ingestion of foreign substances by specialized cells
plasma cell	Specialized cells that develop in the thymus and are responsible for cellular immunity
retrovirus	Type of virus that spreads by using DNA in the body to help it replicate its RNA
sarcoidosis	Inflammation condition with lesions on the lymph nodes and other organs
spleen	Organ of lymph system that filters, stores, removes, blood, and activates lymphocytes
splen(o)	spleen
splenectomy	Removal of the spleen
splenomegaly	Enlarged spleen
suppressor cell	t cell that suppresses B cells and other immune cells
T cells	Specialized cells that develop in the thymus and are responsible for cellular immunity
thym(o)	thymus
thymectomy	Removal of the tyhmus gland
thymocyte	Cell of the thymus gland that can mature into a T cell
thymoma	Tumor of the thymus gland
thymosin	Hormone secreted by the thymus gland that aids in distribution of thymocytes
thymus gland	Soft gland with two lobes that is involved in immune response; located in mediastinum
T lymphocytes	Specialized cells that develop in the thymus and are responsible for cellular immunity
tox(o), toxi, toxico	poison
vaccination vaccine	Injection of an antigen from a different organism to cause active immunity
Western blot	Test primarily used to check for antibodies to HIV in serum
AIDS	acquired immunodenficiency syndrome
ALL	acute lymphocytic leukemia
AML	acute myelogenous leukemia
AZT	Azidothymidine
CLL	chronic lymphocytic leukemia
CML	chronic myelogenous leukemia
CMV	cytomegalovirus
EBV	Epstein-Barr virus
EIS, ELISA	Enzyme-linked immonuosorbent assay
HIV	human immunodeficiency virus
HSV	herpse simples virus
IgA	immunoglobulin A
IgD	immunoglobulin D

IgE	immunoglobulin E
IgG	immunoglobulin G
IgM	immunoglobulin M
PCP	Pneumocystis carinii pneumonia
SLE	systemic lupus erythematosus
ZDV	Zidovudine
abdominocentesis	Incision into the abdomen to remove fluid
absorption	Passing of nutrients into the bloodstream
achalasia	Inability of a muscle, particularly the cardiac sphincter, to relax
achlorhydria	Lack of hydrochloric acid in the stomach
alimentary canal	Muscular tube from the mouth to the anus; digestive tract; gastrointestinal tract
amino acid	Chemical compound that results from digestion of complex proteins
amylase	Enzyme that is part of pancreatic juice and saliva and that begins the digestion of carbohydrates
anal canal	Part of the digestive tract extending from the rectum to the anus
anal fistula	Small opening in the anal canal through which waste matter can leak
anal fistulectomy	Removal of an anal fistula
anastomosis	Surgical union of two hollow structures
ankyloglossia	Conditon of the tongue being partially or completely attached to the bottom of the mouth
an(o)	anus
anorexia	Eating disorder with extreme weight loss
antacid	Agent that neutralizes stomach acid
antidiarrheal	Agent that controls loose, watery stools
antiemetic	Agent that prevents vomiting
antispasmodic	Agent that controls intestinal tract spasms
anus	Place at which feces exit the body
aphagia	Inability to swallow
append(o), appendic(o)	appendix
appendage	Any body part (inside or outside) either subordinate or to a larger part or having no specific central function
appendectomy	Removal of the appendix
appendicitis	Inflammation of the appendix
appendix	Wormlike appendage to the cecum
ascites	Fluid buildup in the abdominal and peritoneal cavities
bil(o), bili	bile
bile	Yellowish-brown to greenish fluid secreted by the liver and stored in the gallbladder; aids in fat digestion
bilirubin	Pigment contained in bile
Billroth's I	Excision of the pylorus
Billroth's II	Resection of the pylorus with the stomach
body	Middle section of the stomach
bowel	Intestine
bucc(o)	cheek
bulimia	Eating disorder with binging and purging
cathartic	Laxative
cec(o)	cecum

cecum	Pouch at the top of the large intestine connected to the bottom of the ileum
celi(o)	abdomen
cheeks	Walls of the oral cavity
cheilitis	Inflammation of the lips
cheiloplasty	Repair of the lips
chol(o), cholo	bile
cholangi(o)	bile vessel
cholangiography	X-ray of the bile ducts
cholangitis	Inflammation of the bile ducts
cholecyst(o)	gallbladder
cholecystectomy	Removal of the gallbladder
cholecystitis	Inflammation of the gallbladder
cholecystography	X-ray of the gallbladder
choledoch(o)	common bile duct
choledocholithotomy	Removal of stones from the common bile duct
cholelithiasis	Gallbladder in the bladder
cholelithotomy	Removal of gallstones
cholelithotripsy	Breaking up or crushing of stones in the body especially gallstones
chyme	Semisolid mass of partially digested food and gastric juices that passes from the stomach to the small intestines
cirrhosis	Liver disease, usually caused by alcoholism
col(o), colon(o)	colon
colectomy	Removal of the colon
colic	Gastrointestinal distress, especially of infants
colitis	Inflammation of the colon
colon	Major portion of the large intestine
colonoscopy	Examination of the colon using an endoscope
colostomy	Creation of an opening from the colon into the abdominal wall
constipation	Difficult or infrequent defecation
Crohn's disease	Type of irritable bowel disease with no ulcers
defecation	Release of feces from the anus
deglutition	Swallowing
diarrhea	Loose, watery stool
digestion	Conversion of food into nutrients for the body and into waste products for release from the body
diverticula	Small pouches in the intestinal walls
diverticulitis	Inflammation of the diverticula
diverticulosis	Condition in which the diverticula trap food or bacteria
duoden(o)	duodenum
duodenal ulcer	Ulcer of the duodenum
duodenum	Top part of the small intestine where chyme mixes with bile, pancreatic juices, and intestinal juice to continue the digestive process
dysentery	Irritation of the intestinal tract with loose stool
dyspepsia	Indigestion
dysphagia	Difficulty is swallowing
emesis	Backward flow from the normal direction
emulsification	Breaking down of fats

enter(o)	intestines
enteritis	Inflammation of the small intestine
enzyme	Protein that causes chemical changes in substances in the digestive tract
epoglottis	Movable flap of tissue that covers the trachea
eructation	Belching
esophag(o)	esophagus
esophagitis	Inflammation of the esophagus
esophagoplasty	Repair of the esophagus
esophagoscopy	Examination of the esophagus with an esophagoscope
esophagus	Part of alimentary canal from the pharynx to the stomach
fatty acid	Acid derived from fat during the digestive process
feces	Semisolid waste that moves through the large intestine to the anus, where it is released from the body
fistula	Abnormal opening in tissue
flatulence	Gas in the stomach or intestines
flatus	Gas in the lower intestinal tract that can be released through the anus
frenulum	Mucous membrane that attaches the tongue to the floor of the mouth
fundus	Upper portion of the stomach
gallbladder	Organ on lower surface of liver; stores bile
gallstones	Calculi in the gallbladder
gastrectomy	Removal of part or all of the stomach
gastric resection	Removal of part of the stomach and repair of the remaining part
gastritis	Inflammation of the stomach
gastr(o)	stomach
gastroenteritis	Inflammation of the stomach and small intestine
gastroscopy	Examination of the stomach using of an endoscope
gloss(o)	tongue
glossectomy	Removal of the tongue
glossitis	Inflammation of the tongue
glossorrhaphy	Suture of the tongue
gluc(o)	glucose
glucose	Sugar found in fruits and plants and in various parts of the body
glyc(o)	sugar
glycogen(o)	glycogen
glycogen	Starch that can be converted into glucose
gums	Fleshy sockets that hold the teeth and aid in chewing
halitosis	Foul mouth odor
hard palate	Hard anterior portion of the palate at the roof of the mouth
hematemesis	Blood in vomit
hematochezia	Red blood in stool
hemorrhoidectomy	Removal of hemorrhoids
hemorrhoids	Swollen, twisted veins in the anus
hepat(o)	liver
hepatic lobectomy	Removal of one ore move lobes of the liver
hepatitis	Inflammation or disease of the liver
hepatomegaly	Enlarged liver
hepatopathy	Liver disease

hiatal hernia	Protrusion of the stomach through an opening in the diaphragm
hyperbilirubinemia	Excessive bilirubin in the blood
icterus	Jaundice
ile(o)	ileum
ileitis	Inflammation of the ileum
ileostomy	Creation of an opening into the ileum
ileus	Intestinal blockage
intussusception	Prolapse of an intestinal part into a neighboring part
jaundice	Excessive bilirubin in the blood causing yellowing of the skin
jejun(o)	jejunum
jejunum	Middle section of the small intestine
labi(o)	lip
large intestine	Passageway in intestinal tract for waste received from small intestine to be excreted through the anus; alos, place where water reabsorption takes place
laxative	Agent that softens stool to relieve constipation
lingu(o)	tongue
lingual tonsils	Two mounds of lymph tissue at the back of the tongue
lipase	Enzyme contained in pancreatic juice
lips	Two muscular folds formed around the outside boundary of the mouth
liver	Organ important in digestive and metabolic functions; secretes bile
liver biopsy	Removal of a small amount of liver tissue to examine for disease
mastication	Chewing
melena	Old blood in the stool
mesentery	Membranous tissue that attaches small and large intestines to the muscular wall at the dorsal part of the abdomen
mouth	Cavity in the face in which food and water is ingested
nausea	Sick feeling in the stomach
obesity	Abnormal accumulation of fat in the body
or(o)	mouth
palatine tonsils	Mounds of tissue on either side of the pharynx
pancreas	Digestive organ that secretes digestive fluids; endocrine gland that regulates blood sugar
pancreat(o)	pancreas
pancreatectomy	Removal of the pancreas
pancreatitis	Inflammation of the pancreas
papilla (pl. papillae)	Tiny projection on the superior surface of the tongue that contains taste buds
paracentesis	Incision into the intestinal tract
parotitis, parotiditis	Inflammation of the parotid gland
pepsin	Digestive enzyme of gastric juice
peptic ulcer	Sore on the mucous membrane if the digestive system; stomach ulcer or gastric ulcer
perisalsis	Coordinated, rhythmic contractions of smooth muscle that force food through the digestive tract
periton(eo)	peritoneum
peritoneoscopy	Examination of the abdominal cavity using a peritoneoscope
peritonitis	Inflammtion of the peritoneum
pharyng(o)	pharynx

polypectomy	Removal of polyps
polyposis	Condition with polyps, as in the intestines
proct(o)	anus, rectum
proctitis	Inflammation of the rectum and anus
proctoplasty	Repair of the rectum and anus
proctoscopy	Examination of the rectum and anus using a proctoscope
pylor(o)	pylorus
pylorus	Narrowed bottom part of the stomach
rect(o)	rectum
rectum	Bottom portion of large intestine; connected to anal canal
reflux	Backward flow from the normal direction
regurgitation	Backward flow from the normal direction
rugae	Folds in stomach lining
salvia	Fluid secreted by salivary glands
salivary glands	Glans in the mouth that secrete fluids that aid in breaking down food
sial(o)	saliva, salivary glands
sialaden(o)	salivary glands
sialoadenitis	Inflammation of the salivary glands
simoid(o)	simoid colon
sigmoid colon	S-shaped part of large intestine connecting at the bottom to the rectum
simoidoscopy	Examination of the sigmoid colon using a sigmoidoscope
small intestine	Twenty-foot long tube that continues the process of digestion started in the stomach; place where most absorption takes place
soft palate	Soft posterior part of the palate in the mouth
steat(o)	fats
steatorrhea	Fat in the blood
stomat(o)	mouth
stomach	Large sac between the esophagus and small intestine; place where food is broken down
stool	Feces
throat	Pharynx
tongue	Fleshy part of the mouth that moves food during mastication
ulcerative colitis	Inflammation of the colon with ulcers
uvula	Cone-shaped projection hanging down from soft palate
villus (pl. villi)	Tiny fingerlike projection on the lining of the small intestine with capillaries through which digested nutrients are absorbed into the bloodstream and lymphatic system
volvulus	Intestinal blockage caused by the intestine twisting on itself
ALT, AT	alanine transaminase
AST	aspartic acit transaminase
BE	barium enema
BM	bowel movement
EGD	esophagogastroduedenoscopy
ERCP	endoscopic rertograde cholangiopancreatography
GERD	gastroesophageal reflux disease
GI	gastrointestinal
IBD	inflammatory bowel disease

IBS	irritable bowel syndrome
NG	nosogastric
NPO	nothing by mouth (Latin nul per os)
SGOT	serum glutamic oxaloacetic transaminase
SGPT	serum glutamic pyruvic transaminase
TPN	total parenteral nutrition
UGI(S)	upper gastrointestinal (series)
acidosis	Abnormal release of ketones in the body
acromegaly	Abnormally enlarged features resulting from a pituitary tumor and hypersecretion of growth hormone
Adam's apple	Protrusion in the neck caused by a fold of thyroid cartilage
Addison's disease	Inderactivity of the adrenal glands
aden(o)	gland
adenectomy	Removal of a gland
adenohyophysis	Anterior lobe of the pituitary gland
adren(o), adrenal(o)	adrenal glands
adrenal cortex	Outer portion of the adrenal gland; helps control metabolism, inflammation, sodium and potassium retention, and effects of stress
adrenalectomy	Removal of an adrenal gland
adrenaline	Epinerphrine; secreted by adrenal medulla
adrenal medulla	Inner portion of adrenal glands; releases large quanties of hormones during stress
adrenocorticotropic hormone (ACTH)	Hormone secreted by anterior pituitary; involved in the control of the adrenal cortex
aldosterone	Hormone secreted by adrenal cortex; mineralocorticoid; affects electrolyte and fluid balance
alpha cells	Specialized cells that produce glucagon in the pancreas
androgen	Any male hormone, such as testosterone
antidiuretic hormone (ADH)	Posterior pituitary hormone that increases water reabsorption; decreases urine output
antihyperglycemic	Agent htat lowers blood glucose
antihyopglycemic	Agent that raised blood glucose
beta cells	Specialized cells that produce insulin in the pancreas
blood sugar, blood glucose	Test for glucose in blood
calcitonin	Hormone secreted by the thyroid gland and othe endocrine glands; help control blood calcium levels
catecholamines	Hormones, such as epinephrine, released in response to stress
corticosteroids	Steroids produced by the adrenal cortex
cortisol	Hydrocortisone
Cushing's syndrome	Group of symptoms caused by overactivity of the adrenal glands
diabetes	Endocrine disorder with abnormally low levels of insulin; also known as insulin-dependent diabetes mellitus (IDDM)
diabetes	Disease caused by failure of the body to recognize insulin that is present or by abnormally low leve of insulin; also known as noninsulin-dependent diabetes mellitus (NIDDM); usually adult onset
diabetes insipidus	Condition caused by hyposecretion of anditiuretic hormone
diabetes mellitus	Endocrine disorder with abnormally low levels of insulin; also known as insulin-dependent diabetes mellitus (IDDM)

diabetes mellitus	Disease caused by failure of the body to recognize insulin that is present or by abnormally low leve of insulin; also known as noninsulin-dependent diabetes mellitus (NIDDM); usually adult onset
diabetic nephropathy	Kidney disease due to diabetes
diabetic neuropathy	Loss of sensation in the extremities due to diabetes
diabetic retinopathy	Gradual loss of vision due to diabetes
ductless gland	Endocrine gland
dwarfism	Abnormally stunted growth caused by hyposecretion of growth hormone, congenital lack of a thyroid gland, or genetic defect
electrolyte	Any substance that conducts electricity and is decomposed by it
endocrine gland	Gland that secretes substances into the bloodstream instead of into ducts
epinephrine	Hormone released by the adrenal medulla in response to stress; adrenaline
exocrine gland	Any gland that releases substances through ducts to a specific location
exophthalmos	Abnormal protrusion of the eyes typical of Grave's disease
fasting blood sugar	Test for glucose in blood following a fast for 12 hours
follicle-stimulating hormone (FSH)	Hormone released by the anterior pituitary to aid in production of ova and sperm
gigantism	Abnormally fast and large growth caused by hypersecretion of growth hormone
gland	Any organized mass of tissue secreting or excreting substances
gluc(o)	glucose
glucogan	Hormone released by the pancreas to increase blood sugar
glucocorticoid	Hormone released by the adrenal cortex
glucose tolerance test (GTT)	Blood test for body's ability to metabolize carbohydratyes; taken after 12-hour fast, then repeated every hour for 4 to 6 hours after ingestion of a sugar solution
glucosuria	Glucose in the urine
glyc(o)	glycogen
glycogen	Converted glucose stored in the liver for future use
glycosuria	Glucose in the urine
goiter	Abnormal enlargement of the thyroid gland as a result of its overactivity or lack of iodine in the diet
gonad(o)	sex glands
Grave's disease	Overactivity of the thyroid gland
growth hormone (GH)	Hormone released by anterior pituitary
hirsutism	Abnormal hair growth due to an excess of androgens
hormone	Substance secreted by glands and carried in the bloodstream to various parts of the body
hormone replacement therapy (HRT)	Ingestion of hormones to replace missing or low levels of needed hormones
hyperadrenalism	Overactivity of the adrenal glands
hyperparathyroidism	Overactivity of the parathyroid glands
hypersecretion	Abnormally high secretion, as from a gland
hyperthyroidism	Overactivity of the thyroid gland
hypoadrenalism	Underactivity of the adrenal gland
hypoglycemia	Abnormally low level of glucose in the blood
hypoglycemic	Agent that lowers blood glucose
hypoparathyroidism	Underactivity of the parathyroid glands
hypophysectomy	Removal of the pituitary gland

hyposecretion	Abnormally low secretion, as from a gland
hypothalamus	Gland in the nervous system that releases hormones to aid in regulating pituitary hormones
hypothyroidism	Underactivity of the thyroid gland
inhibiting	Preventin the secretion of other hormones
insulin	Substance released by the pancreas to lower blood sugar; helps transport glucose to cells and decrease blood sugar
insulin-dependent diabetes mellitus	Endocrine disorder with abnormally low levels of insulin; also known as insulin-dependent diabetes mellitus (IDDM)
islets of Langerhans	Specialized cells in the pancreas that release insulin and glucagon
isthmus	Narrow band of tissue connecting the two lobes of the thyroid gland
ketoacidosis	Condition of high acid levels caused by the abnormal release of ketones in the body
ketosis	Condition caused by the abnormal release of ketones in the body
luteinizing hormone (LH)	Hormone release to aid in maturation of ova and ovulation
melanocyte-stimulating hormone (MSH)	Hormone released by the pituitary gland
melatonin	Hormone released by the pineal gland; affects sexual function and sleep patterns
mineralocorticoid	Steroid secreted by adrenal cortex
myxedema	Advanced adult hypothyroidism
neurohyophysis	Posterior lobe of pituitary gland
noninsulin-dependent diabetes mellitus (NIDDM)	Disease caused by failure of the body to recognize insulin that is present or by abnormally low leve of insulin; also known as noninsulin-dependent diabetes mellitus (NIDDM); usually adult onset
norepinephrine	Hormone secreted by adrenal medulla
ovary	One of two female reproductive glands that secrete hormones in the endocrine system
oxytocin	Hormones released by the posterior pituitray gland to aid in uterine contractions and lactation
pancrease	Gland of both the endocrine system (blood sugar control) and the digestive system (as an exocrine gland)
pancreat(o)	pancreas
pancreatectomy	Removal of the pancreas
pancreatitis	Inflammation of the pancreas
parathormone (PTH)	Parathroid hormone
parathyroid(o)	parathyroid
parathyroidectomy	Removal of one or more of the parathyroid glands
parathyroid gland	One of four glands located adjacent to the thyroid gland on its dorsal surface that help maintain levels of blood calcium
parathyroid hormone	Hormone released by parathyroid glands help raise blood calcium levels
pineal gland	Gland located above pituitary gland; secretes melatonin
pituitary gland	Major endocrine gland; secretes hormones essential to metabolic functions
polydipsia	Excessive thirst
polyuria	Excessive amount of water in the urine
postprandial blood sugar	Test glucose in blood, usually about two hours after a meal
radioactive immunoassay (RIA)	Test for measuring hormone levels in plasma; taken after radioactive solution is ingested
radioactive iodine therapy	Use of radioactive iodine to eliminate thyroid tumors

radioactive iodine uptake	Test for how quickly the thyroid gland pulls in ingested iodine
receptor	Part of a target cell with properties compatible with a particular substance (hormone)
releasing	Allowing secretion of other hormones
somatotrophic hormone (STH)	Hormone secreted by anterior pituitary glands; important in growth and development
steroid	A hormone or chemical substance released by several endocrine glands or manufactured in various medications
suprarenal gland	Adrenal gland
sympathomimetic	Mimicking functions of th esympathetic nervous system
syndorme of inappropiate ADH (SIADH)	Excessive secretion of antidiuretic hormone
target cell	Cell with receptors that are compitable with specific hormones
testis, testicle	One of two male organs that secretes hormones in the endocrine system
tetany	Muscle paralysis, usually due to decreased levels of ionized calcium in the blood
thymectomy	Removal of the thymus gland
thymus gland	Gland that is part of the immune system as well as part of the endocrine system; aids in the maturation of T and B cells
thyr(o) thyroid(o)	thyroid gland
thyroidectomy	Removal of the thyroid
thyroid function test or study	Test for levels for TSH, T3 and T4 in blood plasma to determine thyroid function
thyroid gland	Gland with two lobes located on either side of the trachea; helps control blood calcium levels and metabolic function
thyroid scan	Imaging test for thyroid abnormalities
thyroid-stimulating hormone (TSH)	Hormone secreted by anterior pituitary gland; stimulates release of thyroid hormones
thyrotoxicosis	Overactivtiy of the thyroid gland
thyroxine (T4)	Compound found in or manufactured for thyroid gland; helps regulate metabolism
triiodothyronine (T3)	Thyroid hormone that stimulates growth
Type I diabetes	Endocrine disorder with abnormally low levels of insulin; also known as insulin-dependent diabetes mellitus (IDDM)
Type II diabetes	Disease caused by failure of the body to recognize insulin that is present or by abnormally low leve of insulin; also known as noninsulin-dependent diabetes mellitus (NIDDM); usually adult onset
urine sugar	Test for diabetes; determined by presence of ketones or sugar in urine
vasopressin	Hormone secreted by pituitary gland; raises blood pressure
virilism	Condtion with excessive androgen production, often resulting in the appearance of mature male characteristics in young children
ACTH	adrenocorticotropic hormone
ADH	antidiuretic hormone
CRH	corticotropin-releasing hormone
DM	diabetes mellitus
FSH	follicle-stimulating hormone
GH	growth hormone
GTT	glucose tolerance test
HCG	human chorionic gonadotropin
IDDM	insulin-dependent diabetes mellitus

LH	luteinizing hormone
MSH	melanocyte stimulating hormone
NIDDM	noninsulin-dependent diabetes mellitus
PRL	prolactin
PTH	parathyroid hormone, parathormone
STH	somatotropin hormone
TSH	thyroid-stimulating hormone
aerotitis media	Inflammation of the middle ear caused by air pressure changes; as in air travel
anacusis	Loss of hearing
aphakia	Absence of lens
asthenopia	Weakness of the ocular or ciliary muscle that causes the eyes to tire easily
astigmatism	Distortion of sight because of lack of focus of light rays at one point on the retina
audi(o), audit(o)	hearing
audiogram	Graph that plots the acoustic frequencies being tested
audiologist	Specialist in evaluating hearing function
audiometry	Measurement of acoustic frequencies using an audiometer
auditory ossicles	Three specially shaped bones in the middle ear that anchor the eardrum to the tympanic cavity and that transmit vibrations to the inner ear
aur(o), auricul(o)	hearing
auricle	Funnel-like structure leading from the external ear to the external auditory meatus; also called pinna
blephar(o)	eyelid
blepharitis	Inflammation of the eyelid
blepharochalasis	Loss of elasticity of the eyelid
blepharoplasty	Surgical repair of the eyelid
blepharoptosis	Drooping of the eyelid
blepharospasm	Involuntary eyelid movement; excessive blinking
blindness	Loss or absences of vision
cataract	Cloudiness of the lens of the eye
cerumin(o)	wax
chalazion	Nodular inflammation that usually forms on the eyelid
cholesteatoma	Fatty cyst within the middle ear
choroid	Thin posterior membrane in the middle layer of the eye
ciliary body	Thick anterior membrane in the middle layer of the eye
cochle(o)	cochlea
cochlea	Snail-shaped structure in the inner ear that contains the organ of Corti
cones	Specialized receptor cells in the retina that perceive color and bright light
conjunctiv(o)	conjunctiva
conjunctive (pl. conjunctivae)	Mucous membrane lining of the eyelid
conjunctivitis	Inflammation of the conjunctiva of the eyelid
contact lenses	Corrective lenses worn on the surface of the eye
cor(o), core(o)	pupil
corne(o)	cornea
cornea	Transparent anterior section of the eyeball that bends light in a process called refraction

cryoretinopexy	Fixing of a torn retina using extreme cold
cycl(o)	ciliary body
dacry(o)	tears
dacryoadenitis	Inflammation of the lacrimal glands
dacryocystectomy	Removal of a lacrimal sac
dacryocystitis	Inflammation of a tear duct
deafness	Loss or absence of hearing
decibel	Measure of the intensity of sound
dermatochalasis	Loss of elasticity of the eyelid
diopter	Unit of refracting power of a lens
diplopia	Double vision
ear	Organ of hearing
eardrum	Oval, semitransparent membrane that moves in response to sound waves and produces vibrations
endolymph	Fluid inside the membranous labyrinth important to hearing and equilibrium
enucleation	Removal of an eyeball
epiphora	Excessive tearing
equilibrium	Sense of balance
esotropia	Deviation of one eye inward
eustachian tube	Tube that connects the middle ear to the pharynx
exophthalmos, exophthalmus	Abnormal protrusion of the eyeballs
exotropia	Deviation of one eye outward
eye	Organ of sight
eyebrow	Clump of hair, usually about 1/2-inch above the eye, that helps to keep foreign particles from entering the eye
eyelashes	Group of hairs protruding from the end of the eyelid; helps to keep foreign particles from entering the eye
eyelid	Moveable covering over the eye
farsightedness	Hyperopia
fovea centralis	Depression in the center of the macula lutea; perceives sharpest images
glaucoma	Any various dieseases caused by abnomrally high eye pressure
hearing	Ability to perceive sound
hordeolum	Infection of a sebaceous gland of the eyelid; sty
hyperopia	Focusing behind the retina causing vision distortion; farsightedness
incus	One of three auditory ossicles; the anvil
ir(o), irid(o)	iris
iridectomy	Removal of part of the iris
iridotomy	Incision into the iris to relieve pressure
iris	Colored part of the eye that contains muscles that expand and contract in response to light
iritis	Inflammation of the iris
kerat(o)	cornea
keratitis	Inflammation of the cornea
keratoplasty	Corneal transplant
labyrinthitis	Inflammation of the labyrinth
lacrim(o)	tears
lacrimal glands	Glands that secret liquid to moisten the eyes and produce tears

lacrimation	Secretion of tears, usually excessively
lens	Colorless, flexible transparent body behind the iris
macula	Inner ear structure containing hairlike sensors that move to maintain equilibrium
macula lutea	Small, yellowish area located in the center of the retina, which has a depression called the fovea centralis
macular degeneration	Gradual loss of vision caused by degeneration of tissue of the macula
malleus	One of the three auditory ossicles; the hammer
mastoid(o)	mastoid process
mastoiditis	Inflammation of the mastoid process
membranous labyrinth	One of two tubes that make up the semicircular canals
Meniere's disease	Elvated pressure within the cochlea
miotic	Agent tha causes the pupil to contract
mydriatic	Agent that causes pupil to dilate
myopia	Foccusing in front of the retina causing vision distorting; nearsightedness
myring(o)	eardrum, middle ear
myringitis	Inflammation of the eardrum
myringotomy	Insertion of a small tube to drain fluid from the ears (particularly of children)
nas(o)	nose
nearsightedness	Myopia
neuroretina	Thick layer of nervous tissue in the retina
nyctalopia	Night blindness
nystagmus	Excessive involuntary eyeball movement
ocul(o)	eye
olfactory organs	Organs at the top of the nasal cavity containing olfactory receptors
ophthalm(o)	eye
ophthalmologist	Medical specialist who diagnoses and treats eye disorders
ophthalmoscopy	Visual examination of the interior of the eye
opt(o), optic(o)	eye
optician	Technician who makes and fits corrective lenses
optic nerve	Nerve that transmit nerve impulses from the eye to the brain
optometrist	Nonmedical specialist who examines the eyes and prescribes lenses
organ of Corti	Structure in the basilar membrane with hairlike receptors that receive and transmit sound waves
osseus labyrinth	One of two tubes that make up the semicircular canals
ossicul(o)	ossicle
otalgia	Pain in the ear
otitis externa	Inflammation of the external ear canal
otitis media	Inflammation of the middle ear
otoliths	Small calcifications in the inner ear that help to maintain balance
otologist	Medical specialist in ear disorders
otoplasty	Surgical reapair of the outer ear
otorrhagia	Bleeding from the ear
otorrhea	Purulent discharge from the ear
otosclerosis	Hardening of bones of the ear
otoscopy	Inspection of the ear using an otoscope
papillae	Small, raised structures that contain taste buds

paracusis	Impaired hearing
perilymph	Liquid secreted by the walls of the osseus labyrinth
phac(o), phak(o)	lens
phacoemulsification	Use of ulrasound to break up an remove cataracts
photophobia	Extreme sensitivity to light
pinkeye	Conjunctivitis
pinna	Auricle
presbyacusis	Age-related hearing loss
prebyopia	Age-related dimished ability to focus or accommodate
pseudophakia	Eye with an implanted lens after cataract surgery
pupil	Black circular center of the eye; opens and closes when muscles in the iris expand and contract in response to light
pupill(o)	pupil
refraction	Process of bending light rays
retin(o)	retina
retina	Oval, light-sensitive membrane in the interior layer of the eye; decodes light waves and transmits information to the brain
retinitis pigmentosa	Progressive, inherited disease with a pigmented spot on the retina and poor night vision
rods	Specialized receptor cells in the retina that perceive black to white shades
scler(o)	white of the eye
sclera 9pl. sclerae	Thick, tough membrane in the outer eye layer; supports the eyeball structure
scleritis	Inflammation of the sclera
scot(o)	darkness
scotoma	Blind spot in vision
semicircular canals	Structures in the inner ear important to equilibrium
sensory receptors	Specialized tissue containing cells that can receive stimuli
sensory system	Organs or tissue that perceive and receive stimuli from the outside or within the body
sight	Ability to see
smell	Ability to perceive odors
stapedectomy	Removal of the stapes to cure otosclerosis
stapes (pl. stapes, stapedes)	One of three auditory ossicles; the stirrup
strabismus	Eye misalignment
sty, stye	Hordeolum
taste	Ability to perceive the qualities of ingested matter
taste buds	Organs that sense the taste of food
taste cells	Specialized receptors cells withing the taste buds
tears	Moisture secreted from the lacrimal glands
tinnitus	Constant ringing or buzzing in the ear
tonometry	Measurement of tension or pressure within the eye
touch	Ability to perceive pressure on the skin
trabulectomy	Removal of part of the trabeculum to allow aqueous humor to flow freely around the eye
trichiasis	Abnormal growth of eyelashes in a direction that causes them rub on the eye
tympan(o)	eardrum, middle ear
tympanic membrane	Eardrum

tympanitis	Inflammation of the eardrum
tympanoplasty	Repair of the eardrum
uve(o)	uvea
uvea	Region of the eye containing the iris, choroid membrane, and ciliary bodies
verigo	Dizziness
vestibule	Bony chamber between the semicircular canal and the cochlea
acc.	accommonodation
AD	right ear
ARMD	age-related macular degeneration
AS	left ear
AU	both ears
D	diopter
dB	decibel
DVA	distance visual activity
ECCE	extracapsular cataract extraction
EENT	eye, ear, nose and throat
ENT	ear, nose, and throat
ICCE	intracapsular cataract cryoextraction
IOL	intracular lens
NVA	near visual acuity
OD	right eye
OM	otitis media
OS	left eye
OU	each eye
PERRLA	pupils equal, round, reactive to light and accommonodation
PE tube	polyethylene ventilating tube (placed in the eardrum)
SOM	serious otitis media
VA	visual acuity
VF	visual field
+	plus/convex
-	minus/concave
acanth(o)	spiny; thorny
actin(o)	light
aer(o)	air; gas
alge, algesi, algio, algo	pain
amyl(o)	starch
andro	masculine
athero	plaque; fatty substance
bacill(i)	bacilli; bacteria
bacteri(o)	bacteria
bar(o)	weight; pressure
bas(o), basi(o)	base
bio, Greek bios, life	life
blasto	immature cells
cac(o)	bad; ill
calc(o), calci(o)	calcium

carcin(o)	cancer
chem(o)	chemical
chlor(o)	chlorine, green
chondrio, chondro	cartilage, grainy, gritty
chore(o)	dance
chrom, chromat chromo	color
chrono	time
chyl(o)	chyle, a digestive juice
chym(o)	chyme, semifluid present during digestion
cine(o)	movement
coni(o)	dust
crin(o)	screte
cry(o)	cold
crypt(o)	hidden; obscure
cyan(o)	blue
cycl(o)	circle; cycle; ciliary body
cyst(o), cysti	bladder, cyst, cystic duct
cyt(o)	cell
dextr(o)	right, toward the right
dips(o)	thirst
dors(o), dorsi	back
dynamo	force; energy
echo	reflected sound
electr(o)	electricity; electric
eosin(o)	red; rosy
ergo	work
erythr(o)	red, redness
esthesio	sensation, perception
ethmo	ethmoid bone
etio	cause
fibr(o)	fiber
fluor(o)	light; luminous; fluorine
fungi	fungus
galact(o)	milk
gen(o)	producing; being born
gero; geront(o)	old age
gluco	glucose
glyco	sugars
gonio	angle
granulo	granular
gyn(o), gyne, gyneco	women
home(o), homo	same; constant
hydr(o)	hydrogen, water
hypn(o)	sleep
iatr(o)	physician; treatment
ichthy(o)	dry; scaly; fish

idio	distinct; unknown
immun(o)	safe; immune
kal(i)	potassium
karyo	nucleus
ket(o), keton(o)	ketone; acetone
kin(o), kine	movement
kinesi(o), kineso	motion
kyph(o)	humpback
lact(o), lacti	milk
latero	lateral, to one side
lepto	light, frail, thin
leuk(o)	white
lip(o)	fat
lith(o)	stone
log(o)	speech, words, thought
lys(o)	dissolution
macr(o)	large; long
medi(o)	middle; medial plane
meg(a), megal(o)	large; million
melan(o)	black; dark
mes(o)	middle; median
micr(o)	small; one-millionth; tiny
mio	smaller; less
morph(o)	structure; shape
narco	sleep; numbness
necr(o)	death; dying
noct(i)	night
normo	normal
nucle(o)	nucleus
nyct(o)	night
oncho, onco	tumor
orth(o)	straight; normal
oxy	sharp; acute; oxygen
pachy	thick
path(o)	disease
phago	eating; devouring; swallowing
pharmaco	drugs; medicine
phon(o)	sound; voice; speech
phot(o)	light
physi, physio	physical; natural
physo	air; gas; growing
phyt(o)	plant
plasma, plasmo	formative; plasma
poikilo	varied; irregular
pseud(o)	false
pyo	pus

pyreto	fever
pyro	fever; fire; hear
radio	radiation; x-ray; radius
salping(o)	tube
schisto	split
schiz(o)	split; division
scler(o)	hardness; hardening
scolio	crooked; bent
scoto	darkness
sidero	iron
sito	food; grain
somat(o)	body
somn(o), somni	sleep
sono	sound
spasmo	spasm
spher(o)	round; spherical
spir(o)	breath; breathe
squamo	scale; squamous
staphyl(o)	grapelike clusters
steno	narrowness
stere(o)	three-dimensional
strepto	twisted chains; streptococci
styl(o)	peg-shaped
syring(o)	tube
tel(o), tele(o)	distant; end; complete
terato	monster(as a malformed fetus)
therm	heat
tono	tension; pressure
top(o)	place; topical
tox(i), toxico, toxo	poison, toxin
tropho	food; nurtrition
vivi	life
xanth(o)	yellow
xeno	stranger
xer(o)	dry
xiph(o)	sword; xiphoid
zo(o)	life
zym(o)	fermentation; enzyme
a-	without
ab-,abs-	away from
ad-	toward, to
ambi-	both, around
an-	without
ana-	up, toward
ante-	before
anti-	against

apo-	derived. separate
aut(o)-	self
bi-	twice, double
brachy-	short
brady-	slow
cata-	down
circum-	around
co-, col-, com-, con-, cor-	together
contra-	against
de-	away from
di-, dif-, dir-, dis-	not, separated
dia-	through
dys-	abnormal; difficult
ect(o)-	outside
end(o)-	within
epi-	over
eu-	well, good, normal
ex-	out of, away from
exo-	external, on the outside
extra-	without, outside of
hemi-	half
hyper-	above normal; overly
hypo-	below normal
infra-	positioned beneath
inter-	between
intra-	within
iso-	equal, same
mal-	bad; inadequate
meg(a)-, megal(o)-	large
mes(o)-	middle, median
meta-	after
micr(o)-	small, microscopic
mon(o)-	single
multi-	many
olig(o)-	few; little; scanty
pan-, pnat(o)-	all, entire
par(a)-	beside; abnormal; involving two parts
per-	through intensely
peri-	around, about, near
pluri-	several, more
poly-	many
post-	after, following
pre-	before
pro-	before, forward
quadra-, quadri-	four
re-	again, backward

retro-	behind, backward
semi-	half
sub-	less than, under, inferior
super-	more than, above, superior
supra-	above, over
syl-, sym-, syn-, sys-	together
tachy-	fast
trans-	across, through
ultra-	beyond, excessive
un-	not
uni-	one
-ad	toward
-algia	pain
-asthenia	weakness
-blast	immature, forming
-cele	hernia
-cidal	destroying, killing
-cide	destroying, killing
-clasis	breaking
-crine	secreting
-crit	separate
-cyte	cell
-cytosis	condition of cells
-derma	skin
-desis	bingind
-dynia	pain
-ectasia	expansion; dilation
-ectasis	expanding; dilating
-ectomy	removal of
-edema	swelling
-ema	condition
-emesis	vomiting
-emia	blood
-emic	relating to blood
-esthesia	sensation
-form	in the shape of
-gen	producing, coming to be
-genesis	production of
-genic	producing
-globin	protein
-globulin	protein
-gram	a recording
-graph	recording instrument
-graphy	process of recording
-iasis	pathological condition or state
-ic	pertaining to

-ics	treatment, practice, body of knowledge
-ism	condition, disease, doctrine
-itis (pl. -itides)	imflammation
-kinesia	movement
-kinesis	movement
-lepsy	condition of
-leptic	having seizures
-logist	one who practices
-logy	study, practice
-lysis	destroying
-malacia	softening
-mania	obsession
-megaly	enlargement
-meter	measuring device
-metry	measurement
-oid	like, resembling
-oma (pl. -omata)	tumor, neoplasm
-opia	vision
-opsia	vision
-opsy	view of
-osis (pl. -oses)	condition, state, process
-ostomy	opening
-oxia	oxygen
-para	bearing
-parous	producing; bearing
-paresis	slight paralysis
-pathy	disease
-penia	deficiency
-pepsia	digestion
-pexy	fixation, usually done surgically
-phage, -phagia, -phagy	eating, devouring
-phasia	speaking
-pheresis	removal
-phil	attraction; affinity for
-philia	attraction; affinity for
-phobia	fear
-phonia	sound
-phoresis	carrying
-phoria	feeling; carrying
-phrenia	of the mind
-phthisis	wasting away
-phylaxis	protection
-physis	growing
-plakia	plaque
-plasia	formation
-plasm	formation

-plastic	forming
-plasty	surgical repair
-plegia	paraylsis
-plegic	one who is paralyzed
-pnea	breath
-poiesis	formation
-poietin	one that forms
-poietic	forming
-porosis	lessening in density
-ptosis	falling down; drooping
-rrhage	discharging heavily
-rrhagia	heavy discharge
rrhaphy	surgical suturing
-rrhea	a flowing, a flux
-rrhexis	rupture
-schisis	splitting
-scope	instrument for observing
-scopy	use of an instrument for observing
-somnia	sleep
-spasm	contraction
-stalsis	contraction
-stasis	stopping; constant
-stat	agent to maintain a state
-static	maintaining a state
-stenosis	narrowing
-stomy	opening
-tome	cutting instrument, segment
-tomy	cutting operation
-trophic	nutritional
-trophy	nutrition
-tropia	turning
-tropic	turning toward
-trophy	condition of turning toward
-uria	urine
-version	turning

Medical Terminology
Crosswords

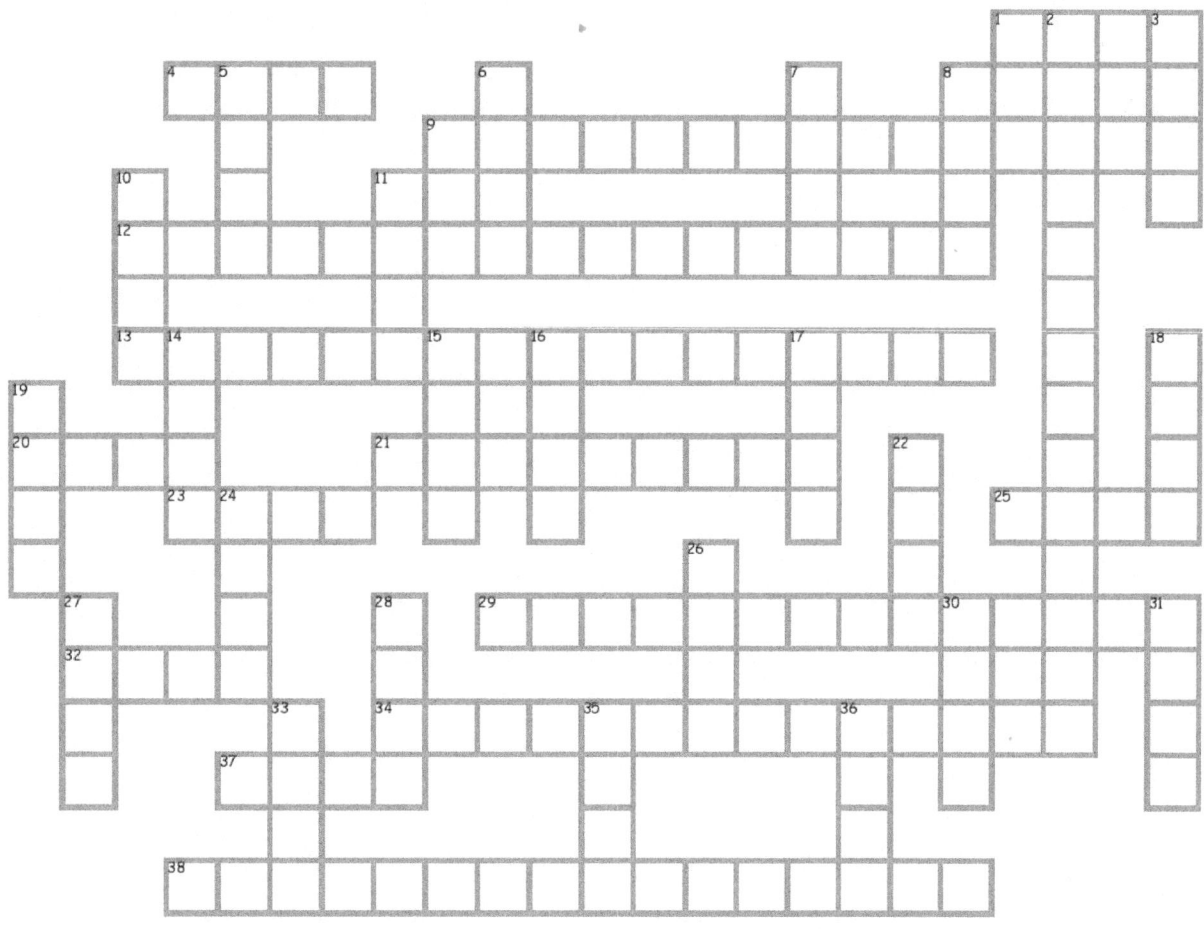

Across

1 agent to maintain a state
4 bio, Greek bios, life
9 voiding (urinating) ____ (VCU, VCUG)
12 acquired ____ syndrome
13 portable device that provides a 24-hour ____.
20 cata-
21 return of a part to its normal position.
23 serum glutamic pyruvic transaminase
25 steat(o)
29 Immature cell formed in bone marrow that becomes ____ into either a red or a white blood cell
32 age-related macular degeneration
34 intracapsular cataract ____
37 bas(o), basi(o)
38 nonsteroidal ____ drug

Down

2 partial ____ time (PTT)
3 chrono
5 insulin-dependent diabetes mellitus
6 cell
7 hernia
8 Middle section of the stomach
10 bil(o), bili
11 quadra-, quadri-
14 Colorless, flexible transparent body behind the iris
15 epi-
16 an(o)
17 producing; being born
18 upper gastrointestinal (series)
19 distinct; unknown
22 serum glutamic oxaloacetic transaminase
24 gastroesophageal reflux disease
26 eye, ear, nose and throat
27 nose
28 extracapsular cataract extraction
30 ir(o), irid(o)
31 coni(o)
33 tachy-
35 blood

36 bad; ill

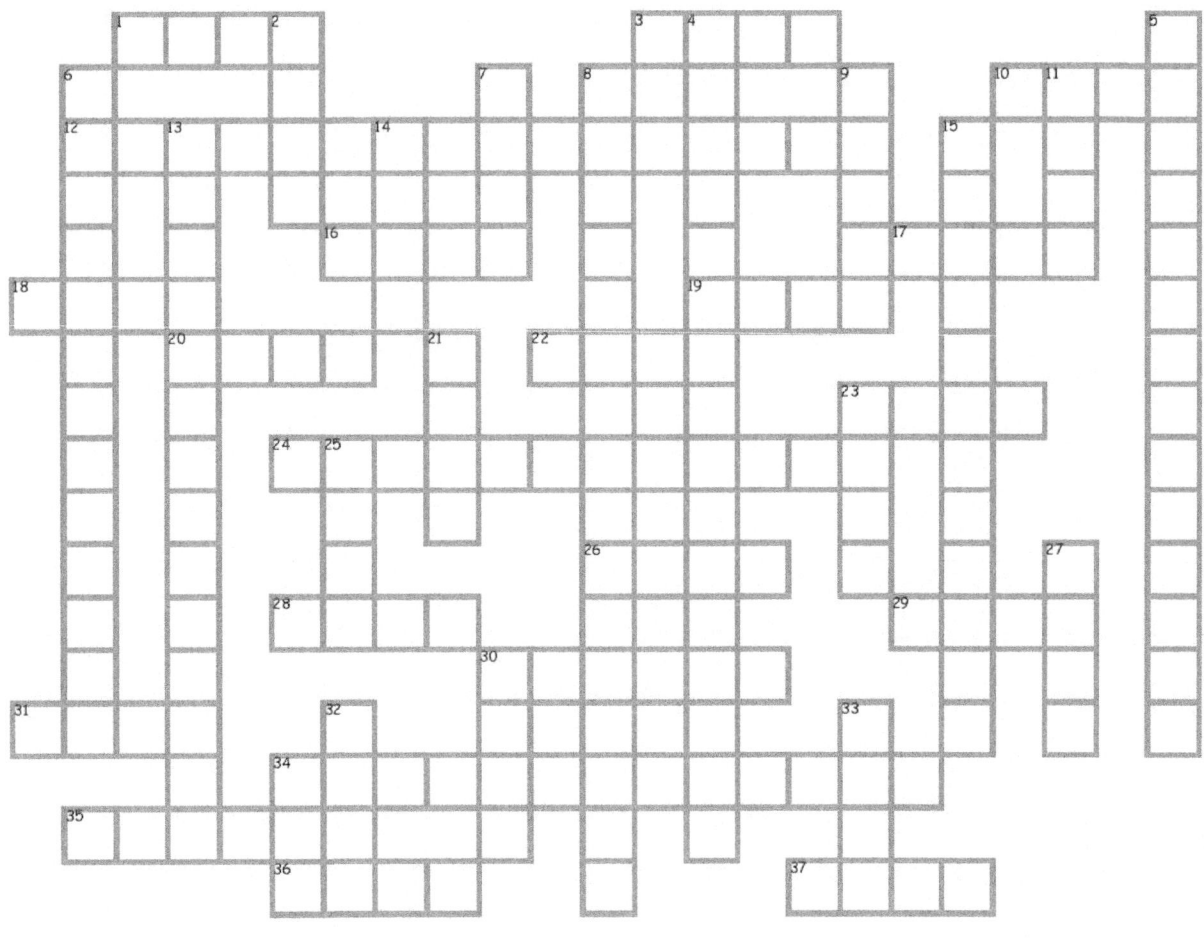

Across

1 phleb(o)
3 fat
10 anterior ridge of the tibia.
12 nonsteriodal ____ drug
16 quadra-, quadri-
17 See verruca flesh-colored growth, sometimes caused by virus; wart
18 mucus
19 blood vessel; duct
20 fungus
22 ost(e), osteo
23 chronic obstructive lung disease
24 Removal of the appendix
26 irid(o)
28 foot
29 opening or hole, particularly in the skin.
30 Sexual intercourse
31 Abnormal sac containing fluid
34 erythrocyte ____ rate (ESR)
35 psych(o), psyche
36 Growth of hard skin, usually on the toes.
37 dry

Down

2 onych(o)
4 bundles of fibers in the ____ septum that transfer charges in the heart's conduction system; also called bundle of His.
5 Nervous system disorder that causes ____, sudden lapses into deep sleep
6 balloon ____
7 pil(o)
8 human ____ virus
9 spinal cords; bone marrow
11 hyperbaric oxygen therapy
13 partial ____ time
14 pod(o)
15 Removal of part of the trabeculum to allow aqueous humor to flow freely around the eye
21 ileum
23 cell
25 hair
27 cephal(o)
30 Abnormally deep sleep with little or no respons to stimuli
32 sebum, sebaceous glands.
33 rhin(o)

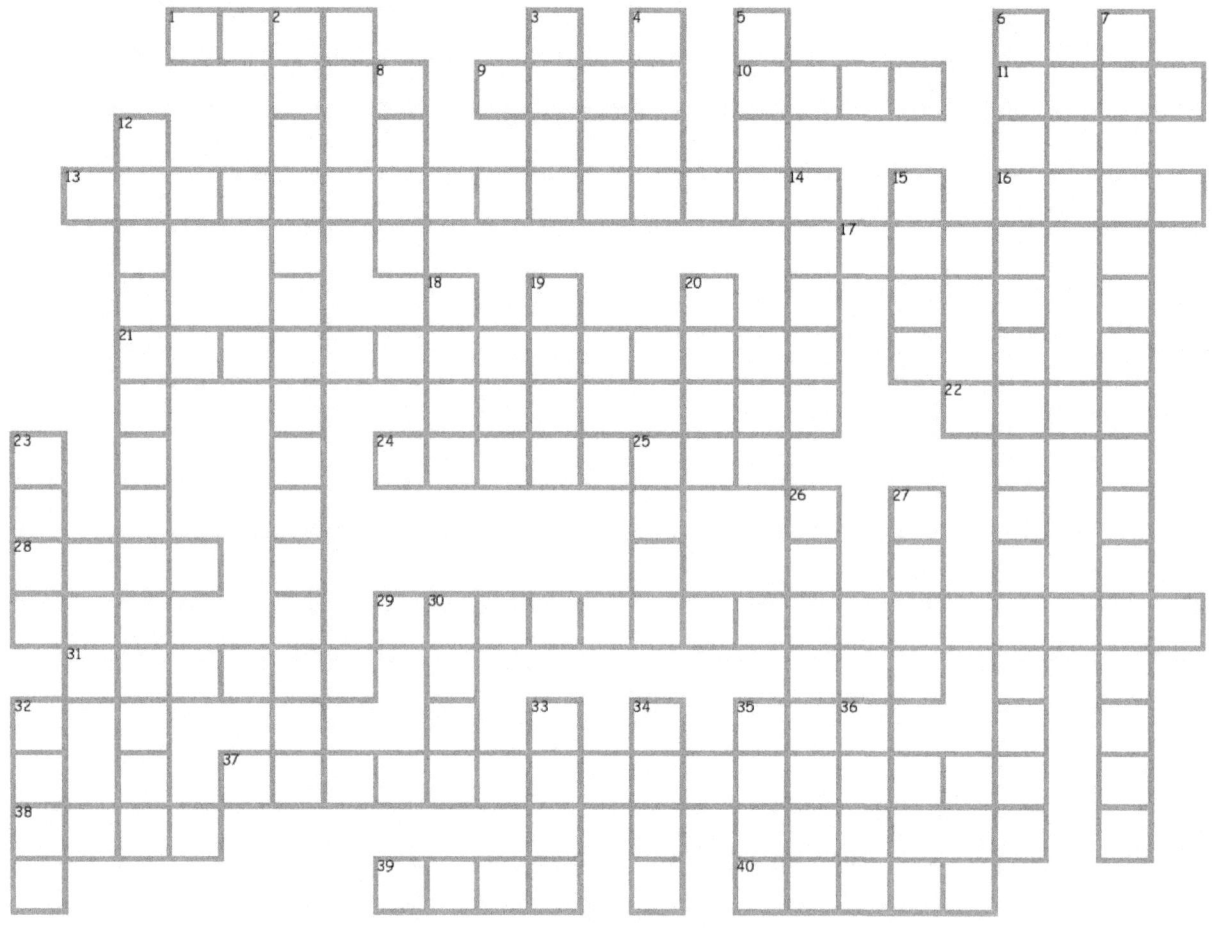

Across

1. Pigment containing iron in hemoglobin
9. fatty
10. ilium
11. psych(o), psyche
13. fatty substance present in animal ____ circulates in the bloodstream, sometimes causing arterial plaque to form.
16. upper gastrointestinal (series)
17. phleb(o)
21. Enzyme-linked ____ assay
22. back, rounded portion of the foot.
24. Inability to produce sperm
28. Abnormal sac containing fluid
29. Muscular tube from the mouth to the anus; digestive tract; ____ tract
31. audi(o), ____)
37. intracorporeal ____ lithotripsy
38. Damage to the skin caused by exposure to heat, chemicals, electricity, radiation, or other skin irritants.
39. dry
40. Ability to see

Down

2. One of the four major divisions of the brain; division that coordinates ____ movement
3. sudden infant death syndrome
4. ost(e),osteo
5. hair
6. human ____ virus (HIV)
7. Agent with ____ properties.
8. pod(o)
12. medication used for heart failure and other ____ problems; acts by dilating arteries to lower blood pressure and makes heart pump easier.
14. first lumbar vertebra, second lumbar vertebra, etc.
15. sebum, sebaceous glands.
18. Specialized receptor cells in the retina that perceive black to white shades
19. opening or hole, particularly in the skin.
20. half
23. cervic(o)
25. mucus
26. adrenocorticotropic hormone
27. blood vessel; duct
30. activated partial thromboplastin time
32. pubis
33. foot
34. dissolution

35 infant respiratory distress syndrome
36 pulmon(o)

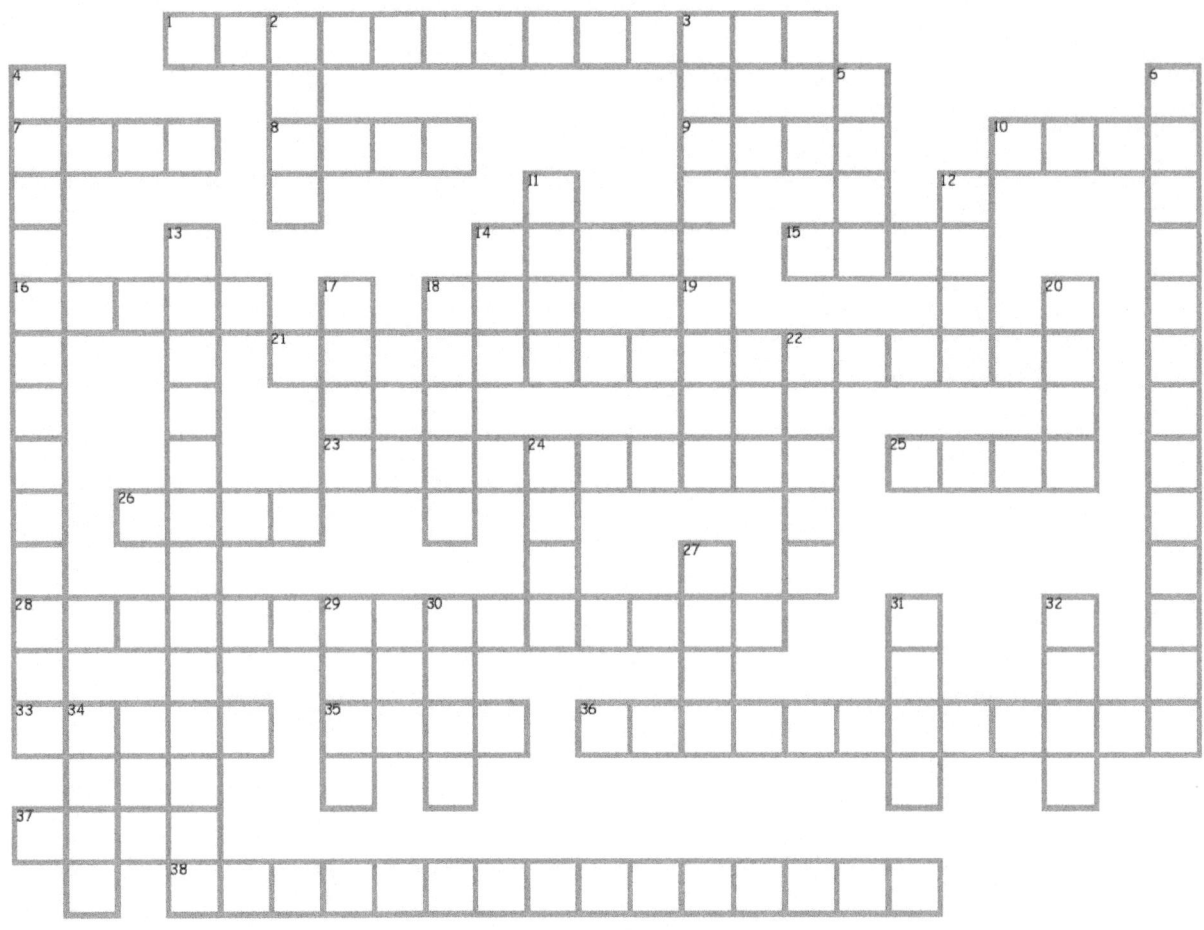

Across

1. lactate ____
7. echocardiogram
8. second cervical vertebra.
9. back, rounded portion of the foot.
10. Damage to the skin caused by exposure to heat, chemicals, electricity, radiation, or other skin irritants.
14. trachel(o)
15. blood vessel; duct
16. Male sex cell that contains chromosomes
21. nonsteriodal ____ drug
23. test that measures heart rate, blood pressure, and other body functions while the patient is exercising on a treadmill.
25. ped(i), pedo
26. fungus
28. proximal ____ joint
33. nonsteroidal anti-inflammatory drug
35. psych(o), psyche
36. Imaginary line that insects the body ____.
37. opening or hole, particularly in the skin.
38. Oval, ____ membrane that moves in response to sound waves and produces vibrations

Down

2. cephal(o)
3. arteriosclerotic heart disease
4. cardiopulmonary ____
5. uln(o)
6. fibrous muscle of internal organs that acts ____.
11. veni, veno
12. foot
13. laboratory test that provides the levels of lipids, ____, and other substances in the blood.
17. proct(o)
18. sweat, sweat glands
19. bottom section of the lung
20. Abnormal sac containing fluid
22. uterus
24. dermat(o)
27. trich(o), trichi
29. Pigment containing iron in hemoglobin
30. pulmon(o)
31. Inflammatory eruption of the skin, occurring in or near sebaceous glands on the face, neck, shoulder, or upper neck.
32. hair
34. serum glutamic oxaloacetic transaminase

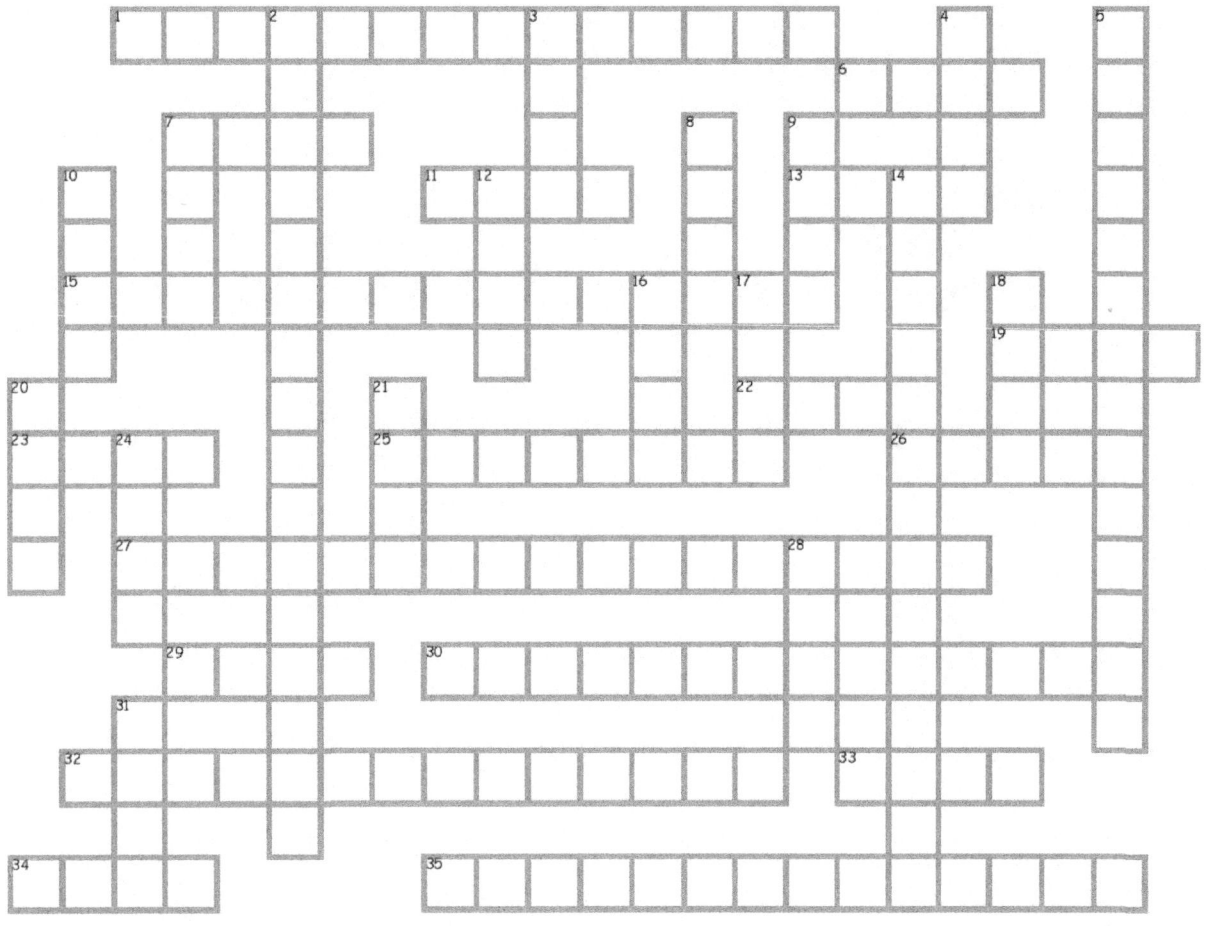

Across

1. Protein produced by T cells and other cells; destroys ____ cells with its antiviral properties
6. serum glutamic oxaloacetic transaminase
7. postitive and expiratory pressure
11. Granulocyte colony-stimulating factor
13. Group of sypmtoms that precede a seizure
15. proximal ____ joint
19. Part of a nerve cell that conducts nerve impulses away from the cell body
22. cata-
23. Two muscular folds formed around the outside boundary of the mouth
25. inflammation of bursa
26. darkness
27. Disease involving overproduction of antibodies that block certain ____; causes muscle weakness
29. an(o)
30. intracapsular cataract ____
32. stationary blood clot in the ____ system, usually found from matter found in the blood.
33. galact(o)
34. Middle portion of the uterus
35. Test of a blood specimen in a culture medium to observe for particular ____

Down

2. intracorporeal ____ lithotripsy
3. acquired immunodeficiency disease
4. Abnormally deep sleep with little or no respons to stimuli
5. Enzyme-linked ____ assay
7. after, following
8. bil(o), bili
9. onych(o)
10. neuroglia
12. chronic obstructive lung disease
14. surgical ____ of a cardiac valve.
16. Manner of walking
17. adult respiratory disease syndrome
18. vagus nerve
20. ileum
21. hyperbaric oxygen therapy
24. Part of the brainstem that controls certain respiratory functions
28. transurethral resection of the prostate
31. continuous ambulatory peritoneal dialysis

Medical Terminology
Word Search

Medical Definitions Word Search Puzzle

```
A U F V P E A P I L Z N A R B B M S S E C O R P D I O L Y T S P V P Q
C F I G L H O Y A V R E O W M W F L C M T S A L C O E T S O G C Q R T
O K S I N I Y M M F W U E D M E L C S U M D E T A I R T S T N I F O O
Q N P E E I I S R X N R R S U J K R D I M U R E T H R O N Q I D B X L
B U M S S N K A I T E O U I S L Y B M R T K W S Q A M E M V D O X I B
P E I X A P C A O S M P S T L H E Q F T V D U X D A B L O T N M P M N
S S S M Q T I N E U O L S I S E S E A E S E I D D O D U O U S S A R
T I S S U E S N Y R D A I R R E G U L A R B O N E S E O L C O A O L E
R S S R Y I W L A J B S F E T Y C O M Y H T V K I P H L I A R P R X T
C F E H L C K T E L A T J L B R S T E A T O O T I G E T K P R S I N S
H F I S H S C A L Y C Y F C S T R O K E Z O R D U B E G J A U I A Y E
S W E A T G L A N D S O T S E H C D W X R O E O E R Y L T D S T S R W
N E V R E N C I T P O D R H I G F G G C C P R R U L Y I U J S N I A Z
U M B I L I C A L C O R D D X X M G U V F H E I L A T E R A L S L J
Q T S E T N I L U B O L G I T N A N J Z T C D E Q J Q L O C A T E D O
```

- ☐ SPINAL CORD
- ☐ NEUROPLASTY
- ☐ LOCATED
- ☐ ABDOMEN
- ☐ TISSUE
- ☐ THROUGHOUT
- ☐ ANTISPASMODIC
- ☐ STEAT(O)
- ☐ -PHYSIS
- ☐ STROKE
- ☐ SCLERITIS
- ☐ SWEAT GLANDS
- ☐ DIURETIC
- ☐ TONSILS
- ☐ FISSURE
- ☐ LARYNX
- ☐ PUPIL
- ☐ FISH, SCALY
- ☐ URETHR(O)
- ☐ ATRIUM
- ☐ UMBILICAL CORD
- ☐ STYLOID PROCESS
- ☐ SEMEN
- ☐ PSORIASIS
- ☐ NODULE
- ☐ PROXIMAL
- ☐ OSTEOCLAST
- ☐ BREAKING
- ☐ STRIATED MUSCLE
- ☐ -POIESIS
- ☐ CHEST
- ☐ LAMINA
- ☐ ANTIGLOBULIN TEST
- ☐ FRACTURE
- ☐ IRREGULAR BONES
- ☐ PED(I), PEDO
- ☐ SURROUNDING
- ☐ CROOKED; BENT
- ☐ CEREBELL(O)
- ☐ RADI(O)
- ☐ WESTERN BLOT
- ☐ OPTIC NERVE
- ☐ CORTISOL
- ☐ THYMOCYTE
- ☐ DIESEASES
- ☐ LATERAL

Medical Definitions Word Search Puzzle

```
G S S E C O R P S U O N I P S A F A I N O T O P Y H P A R G O M M A M
T I B I A U Z E B C T H I S O V I M I M P A W P P S N D P N Y R O S Y
A D R E N A L G L A N D S I L K D I A B E T E S Y I T R E G U R T E M
O T E N D O N X D C J K S T O E N I M E N R O R L S E E C M T H G S O
G N X N Y R A H P Y S E Q I I P E Z T Q I E O D O A H N A A N E N A T
N S I T I T C O R P D U U B H I C Q Y N N L E A P T R A R I C M I E O
Y T K Y O Q U F C U G L M E C S G S E I G S M N E C X L T D P O N R H
R P G G U T I O L F R S E L N I J U R T A O S O L E X E E Z F G I C T
A M H X S S S C Y Q J P J H O O M E S E U H G D I L Q C R Y U L A N I
L X G I S T N O R H P E N P R S P T L T G Z M U S E K T I O V O T I L
V Y D U O I Y M O T O N E T B T D E H N F D H L S T Q O T C Z B R C E
M E R U Z I E S L A M D N A R G R S A C R U M E E A P M I D G I E P L
W E Y P V I S C E R A L P L E U R A P N S W K O S T P Y S Z N N P Z O
C U S H I N G S S Y N D R O M E B O N E S C A N C E L L U L I T I S H
D R A L U C I R T N E V O I R T A U F Y Q S W E A T G L A N D S H W C
```

- ☐ INCREASES
- ☐ NODULE
- ☐ XER(O)
- ☐ CUSHING'S SYNDROME
- ☐ MOUTH
- ☐ OUTSIDE
- ☐ CHOLELITHOTOMY
- ☐ GRAND MAL SEIZURE
- ☐ BRONCHIOL(O)
- ☐ COST(O)
- ☐ INCLUDES
- ☐ LARYNG(O)
- ☐ HYPOTONIA
- ☐ ARTERITIS
- ☐ HEMOGLOBIN
- ☐ ADRENALECTOMY
- ☐ CELLULITIS
- ☐ PHARYNX
- ☐ SWEAT GLANDS
- ☐ SESSILE POLYP
- ☐ RELEASED
- ☐ PERINEUM
- ☐ FISSURE
- ☐ SPINOUS PROCESS
- ☐ AORTA
- ☐ MAMMOGRAPHY
- ☐ PERTAINING TO
- ☐ TENDON
- ☐ SACRUM
- ☐ PERINE(O)
- ☐ EPISI(O)
- ☐ VISCERAL PLEURA
- ☐ MUSCLE
- ☐ PHLEBITIS
- ☐ OPENING
- ☐ PROCTITIS
- ☐ ATRIOVENTRICULAR
- ☐ ATELECTASIS
- ☐ ADRENAL GLANDS
- ☐ BONE SCAN
- ☐ TENOTOMY
- ☐ TIBIA
- ☐ NEPHRON
- ☐ DIABETES

Medical Definitions Word Search Puzzle

```
M Y O C A R D I A L S S S P G F M A Y M O T O H T I L O R H P E N G H G
K I N V I R I L I S M W C D K P S X F B F W U P Y M O T O R U E N Y Y
A I D S Y R V A T T T A C O N T A I N U G F Y I M E T R Y D C U S D P
H M H E B M E N N L I Z A A T J Q Z D L S D H S A N Y S G S L M X R O
U B U A S H O E F R L I X K W O G P G L V D A E O O T I X B E O I O C
P D M I R L M T E N T I S S U E W M E A R R A S R I M S Y L U J V N S
L N V R D H U T O E K Q I F E E Z T R P J H C F N S I O L O Z M R E O
E U A S C R E P Y L M S L U H C K M E L A N I N E N R H Q O I T E P R
M I M A X M A E M K E Z I R Y A E N F B M G D C R E I R V D C L C H E
D F T B O U S C N I A Y O U G T I F K U S I M M M V T W R G R H V K R T
Q T V R A I B V I H E C P N V M G C S L S N B I O R C I P O R T C O S
A F I K G R A J A R A V C C C Z C C S L I U L P U E X C X V U R E S Y
I P Z H C A L C A N E O R L P C L S U A N Y N Y S P O M M A M Y N I H
S X T R K L J T I Q W P M E T E I G F E F N K A Q Y P O Y R A K X S L
F J W A D I F F E R E N T E N V A L V U L I T I S H E R O S D L O C N
```

- ☐ CIRRHOSIS
- ☐ BLOOD
- ☐ CONTAIN
- ☐ LIVER
- ☐ MELANIN
- ☐ TISSUE
- ☐ HYPERTENSION
- ☐ PERICARDIUM
- ☐ FECES
- ☐ NEPHROLITHOTOMY
- ☐ SPIROMETER
- ☐ MUSCLE
- ☐ FURUNCLE
- ☐ -TROPIC
- ☐ SCOT(O)
- ☐ NEUROTOMY
- ☐ BULLA(PL.BULLAE)
- ☐ AIDS
- ☐ MAMM(O)
- ☐ DIARRHEA
- ☐ HYDRONEPHROSIS
- ☐ GM-CSF
- ☐ VIRILISM
- ☐ NECK;CERVIX
- ☐ NERVE IMPULSE
- ☐ ATTACHMENT
- ☐ DIFFERENT
- ☐ FASCIA
- ☐ KARY(O)
- ☐ HYSTEROSCOPY
- ☐ SMELL
- ☐ -METRY
- ☐ VALVULITIS
- ☐ LUMBAR
- ☐ ANUS
- ☐ EYE; SIGHT
- ☐ CALCANE(O)
- ☐ PYELOTOMY
- ☐ ILI(O)
- ☐ NERVOUS
- ☐ MYOCARDIAL
- ☐ COLD SORE
- ☐ ASHD

Medical Definitions Word Search Puzzle

```
L D Y A R W T P S M S U R G E R Y X J U K E L B U O D E C I W T N T C
N E R U Z J K T N E D I O C I T R O C O L A R E N I M A Z R E M E O A
O N X O V L O O Z L F S H O L U B A T E C A P S D A R K N E S S X L R
I S O H C M I H L A E Y C E L L U L I T I S I O I R A B M U L F H I O
T I J A A T B A L N P A E H R R O B E S K J O M S S Q F J D Z N A G T
I T T C A V J L O O L H S I N U S I T I S D M O E I O R N M W Y L U I
T O H T A U O B D C A M O V T X E U S F Y A Y S B X S C M I B U A R D
U M S G R P L E D Y S T N E M U R T S N I Z H B S S O S A N I H T I W
L E E F I A R Y R T M F T K Y M M F X I N C T H L E I P A R Z W I A G
G T D A S M W V X E A A G A S T R O S C O P Y A O S Y F Y R H W O F F
E E N A I X I M M U N I T Y M R B P W I M P A T R L W Q T H C T N T Z
D R N S E P I J Q Y I N T E R L E U K I N A V H T U Y G K W W O N B Z
I R O N I H A M N I O T S Y C L A D I N O L I P N P C Y H R N X M A Z
F N P A N C R E A T I T I S I T I T A T S O R P O M R O I R E T N A I
Z O F N O I T A L L I R B I F L A I R T A H N K C I A I L G O R C I M
```

- MELANOCYTE
- THYM(O)
- OLIGURIA
- PANCREATITIS
- GESTATION
- HYPOXEMIA
- WITHIN
- DEGLUTITION
- SEBORRHEA
- IRON
- PILONIDAL CYST
- STOMACH
- ACETABUL(O)
- ANTERIOR
- LUMBAR
- CONTROLS
- ATRIAL FIBRILLATION
- TETANY
- SINUSITIS
- AMNI(O)
- HYPODERMIS
- IMMUNITY
- SURGERY
- ANTHRACOSIS
- PLASMA
- INSTRUMENT
- EXHALATION
- DARKNESS
- CAROTID
- HEAD
- FALLOPIAN
- MINERALOCORTICOID
- KAPOSI'S SARCOMA
- GASTROSCOPY
- IMPULSES
- INTERLEUKIN
- MICROGLIA
- DENSITOMETER
- TWICE, DOUBLE
- CELLULITIS
- PROSTATITIS
- TAH-BSO
- NASAL BONES

Medical Definitions Word Search Puzzle

```
T Q D V N R R S U P U L F O M R O F D L I M V L E S L U P D S G Q E W
D A H I Y E T N E M E V O M V O N I S O E I A Y L S P R E Y V E A N A
L V L A B R R O S S A N O I T C E S N A E R A S E A C R R S N S U D M
O M E I S R O V R Z O D E R E T L I F E Y A R I E E S A O P O A R O O
C Q G U P I E T O N O N I T U S Q E C N S P T S H H L B P A I E I C L
H X X Z M E L A I U L C E R S U V A G R R R H E A R L N I R G S N R Y
U A D I P O S E T D S B Q U O I F O U E A E O R R R E I T E E I E I D
T R A C H E A V S H U S W K T R P B K X L S G O T O C E U U R D S N N
L C I A A U N B A I I A Y C U H T A Z E R S R H E K A T I N R S U E O
K L J N G M E E T L E N A S A Z M L A S E U A P R U H S T I A E G G C
E O X J E E G X X C G O G R T E L G R U A R P A I E P P A A B V A L M
E L E C T R I C A L I U Y J C E U N B X D E H I E L L E R A M A R A T
K Y J P F C T U Q D V N S A R R M V P M Y K Y D S X A E Y Q U R V N K
O N R G S L N R A S X B P F Y L R A L U C S U M A R T N I W L G T D S
B A D B M U A R Y T I N U M M I L A R U T A N E N T I R E L Y Z N R Q
```

- NOSE
- URINE
- ELECTRICAL
- RADIOACTIVE
- INTRAMUSCULARLY
- CAESAREAN SECTION
- ALPHA CELLS
- LUMBAR REGION
- EPSTEIN-BARR
- PORE
- DYSPAREUNIA
- ALREADY
- ARTHOGRAPHY
- ARTERIES
- PULSE
- TALIPES VALGUS
- BREATHING
- AUDITORY
- MILD FORM OF LUPUS
- COLD
- PACEMAKER
- BURSA
- ANTIGEN
- DIAPHORESIS
- EIS, ELISA
- CONDYLOMA
- URINE SUGAR
- MOVEMENT
- LEUKORRHEA
- RUGAE
- ADIPOSE
- HEEL
- NERVOUS SYSTEM
- LARYNGOPHARYNX
- NATURAL IMMUNITY
- EOSINO
- SURFACE
- PRESSURE
- ENTIRELY
- GRAVE'S DISEASE
- ENDOCRINE GLAND
- FILTERED
- TRACHEA
- ULCERS
- PITUITARY

Medical Terminology
Matching

Medical Definitions Matching

Write the letter corresponding to the correct match in the space provided.

___ 1. carcinoma in situ
___ 2. perisalsis
___ 3. mammoplasty
___ 4. patent ductus arteroosus
___ 5. actin(o)
___ 6. blephar(o)
___ 7. metacarpal
___ 8. spinal cord
___ 9. stratum(pl. strata)
___ 10. cardi(o)
___ 11. arteriography
___ 12. -cide
___ 13. ophthalm(o)
___ 14. -phonia
___ 15. trabulectomy
___ 16. heart transplant
___ 17. plastic surgery
___ 18. extracorporeal shock wave lithotripsy (ESWL)
___ 19. ankle
___ 20. -tropia

A. Plastic surgery to reconstruct the breast, particularly after a mastectomy
B. Ropelike tissue that sits inside the vertebral column and from which spinal nerves extend
C. turning
D. destroying, killing
E. a condition at birth in which the ductus arteriosus, a small duct between the aorta and the pulmonary artery, remains abnormally open.
F. sound
G. Breaking of kidney stones by using shock waves from outside the body
H. implantation of the heart of a person who has just died into a person whose diseased heart cannot sustain life.
I. Removal of part of the trabeculum to allow aqueous humor to flow freely around the eye
J. heart; esophageal opening of the stomach
K. eyelid
L. eye
M. Coordinated, rhythmic contractions of smooth muscle that force food through the digestive tract
N. one of the five bones of the hand between the wrist and the fingers.
O. Localized malignancy that has not spread
P. repair or reconstruction(as of the skin) by means of surgery.
Q. Hinged area between the lower leg bones and the bones of the foot.
R. viewing of a specific artery by x-ray after injection of contrast medium
S. layer of tissue, especially a layer of skin.
T. light

Medical Definitions Matching

Write the letter corresponding to the correct match in the space provided.

___ 1. P
___ 2. LH
___ 3. ringworm
___ 4. lact(o), lacti
___ 5. myxedema
___ 6. LV
___ 7. intrauterine device (IUD)
___ 8. femoral artery
___ 9. esophagus
___ 10. oropharynx
___ 11. thorac(o)
___ 12. spondyl(o)
___ 13. adenoidectomy
___ 14. bacteri(o)
___ 15. trachel(o)
___ 16. neurohyophysis
___ 17. malleus
___ 18. tachy-
___ 19. diaphragm
___ 20. herniated disk

A. luteinizing hormone
B. bacteria
C. fast
D. fungal infection; tinea
E. vertebra
F. Posterior lobe of pituitary gland
G. protrusion of an intervertebral disk into neural canal
H. Contraceptive device consisting of a coil placed in the uterus to block implantation of a fertilized ovum
I. para (live birth)
J. Back portion of the mouth, a division of the pharynx
K. neck
L. One of the three auditory ossicles; the hammer
M. left ventricle
N. Advanced adult hypothyroidism
O. thorax
P. membranous muscle between the abdominal and thoracic cavities that contracts and relaxes during the respiratory cycle.
Q. Part of alimentary canal from the pharynx to the stomach
R. milk
S. removal of the adenoids
T. an artery that supplies blood to the thigh.

Medical Definitions Matching

Write the letter corresponding to the correct match in the space provided.

___ 1. tympanitis
___ 2. herniated disk
___ 3. pro-
___ 4. chlor(o)
___ 5. -trophic
___ 6. fulguration
___ 7. MCHC
___ 8. carotid artery
___ 9. hyperthyroidism
___ 10. atrioventricular block
___ 11. cardiac arrest
___ 12. natural immunity
___ 13. pruritus
___ 14. hormone
___ 15. urostomy
___ 16. ophthalm(o)
___ 17. expectorants
___ 18. Grave's disease
___ 19. purpura
___ 20. ketosis

A. Overactivity of the thyroid gland
B. before, forward
C. agents that promote the coughing and expelling of mucus.
D. artery that transport oxygenated blood to the head and neck
E. Condition caused by the abnormal release of ketones in the body
F. itching
G. Inflammation of the eardrum
H. Condition with multiple, tiny hemorrhages under the skin
I. chlorine, green
J. eye
K. nutritional
L. protrusion of an intervertebral disk into neural canal
M. destruction of tissue using electric sparks.
N. mean corpuscular hemoglobin concentration
O. sudden stopping of the heart; also called asystole.
P. Establishment of am opening in the abdomen to the exterior of the body for the release of urine
Q. Substance secreted by glands and carried in the bloodstream to various parts of the body
R. heart block; partial or complete blockage of the electrical impulses from the atrioventricular node.
S. Inherent resistance to disease found in a species, race, family group, or certain individuals
T. Overactivity of the thyroid gland

Medical Definitions Matching

Write the letter corresponding to the correct match in the space provided.

___ 1. splen(o)
___ 2. flutter
___ 3. SV
___ 4. orchidectomy
___ 5. receptor
___ 6. duodenal ulcer
___ 7. -plasm
___ 8. AS
___ 9. pelvimetry
___ 10. col(o), colon(o)
___ 11. thalassemia
___ 12. BCP
___ 13. metacarp(o)
___ 14. esophagus
___ 15. sperm(o) spermat(o)
___ 16. shingles
___ 17. histi(o), histo
___ 18. thoracic vertebrae
___ 19. croup
___ 20. HIV

A. metacarpal
B. acute respiratory syndrome in children or infants accompanied by seal-like coughing.
C. formation
D. Ulcer of the duodenum
E. viral disease affecting peripheral nerves and caused by herpes zoster.
F. Part of alimentary canal from the pharynx to the stomach
G. twelve vertebrae of the chest area.
H. biochemistry panel
I. aortic stenosis
J. Removal of a testicle
K. stroke volume
L. sperm
M. Measurement of the pelvis during pregnancy
N. Hereditary disorder characterized by inability to produce sufficient hemoglobin
O. tissue
P. regular but very rapid heartbeat.
Q. Tissue or organ that receives nerve impulses
R. human immunodeficiency virus
S. spleen
T. colon

Medical Definitions Matching

Write the letter corresponding to the correct match in the space provided.

___ 1. VT
___ 2. arteri(o) arter(o)
___ 3. seg
___ 4. afterbirth
___ 5. arthr(o)
___ 6. -poiesis
___ 7. cardiotonic
___ 8. calcane(o)
___ 9. vesicle
___ 10. glyco
___ 11. red blood cell count
___ 12. colp(o)
___ 13. stress test
___ 14. ventriculgram
___ 15. adrenal medulla
___ 16. -trophy
___ 17. tine test
___ 18. VF
___ 19. immunoglobulin
___ 20. auricle

A. Measurement of red blood cells in a cubic millimeter of blood
B. artery
C. ventricular tachycardia
D. Placenta and membranes that are expelled from the uterus afterbirth
E. small, raised sac on the skin containing fluid.
F. visual field
G. medication for congestive heart failure; increases the force of contractions of the myocardium.
H. x-ray of a ventricle taken after injection of a contrast medium.
I. test for tuberculosis in which a small dose of tuberculin is injected into a series of sites within a small space with a tine (instrument that punctures the surface of the skin).
J. vagina
K. test that measures heart rate, blood pressure, and other body functions while the patient is exercising on a treadmill.
L. Type of antibody
M. Inner portion of adrenal glands; releases large quanties of hormones during stress
N. heel
O. sugars
P. Funnel-like structure leading from the external ear to the external auditory meatus; also called pinna
Q. joint; articulation
R. condition of turning toward
S. segmented mature white blood cells
T. formation

Medical Terminology
Quiz and Test

Medical Definitions Quiz

Circle the letter of the Answer that corresponds to the displayed Question Combining Forms.

1. alge, algesi, algio, algo
    - A. Reversal of a vasectomy
    - B. phenylketonuria
    - C. obsession
    - D. pain

2. lung
    - A. One of two organs of respiration (left lung and right lung) in the thoracic cavity where oxyegenation of blood takes place
    - B. Tissue or organ that receives nerve impulses
    - C. thick
    - D. Inflammation of the kidneys

3. lumen
    - A. Urinary incontinence
    - B. Belching
    - C. hysterosalpingography
    - D. channel inside an artery through which blood flows.

4. nail
    - A. Removal of a lacrimal sac
    - B. Most malignant type of glioma
    - C. thin layer of keratin that covers the distal portion of fingers and toes.
    - D. Abnormally high secretion, as from a gland

5. bronchus (pl. bronchi)
    - A. esophagus
    - B. measuring device
    - C. one of the two airways from the trachea to the lungs.
    - D. insertion of a tube through the nose or mouth, pharynx, and larynx and into the trachea to establish an airway.

6. ulna
    - A. larger bone of the forearm
    - B. nail
    - C. complete blood count
    - D. Rare, congenital condition causing either partial or total lack of pigmentation.

7. otitis externa

A. Test glucose in blood, usually about two hours after a meal

B. Inflammation of the external ear canal

C. removal of a bunion

D. Changing of a liquid, especially blood, into a semi-solid

8. ovari(o)

   A. Common group of automated tests run on one blood sample

   B. channel inside an artery through which blood flows.

   C. Blood test for prostate cancer

   D. ovary

9. dia-

   A. Progressive, inherited disease with a pigmented spot on the retina and poor night vision

   B. through

   C. inflammation of the epiglottis

   D. Passageway at back of mouth for air and food; throat

10. diaphragm

    A. dyspnea on exertion

    B. Fibrous substance that forms the body's supportive framework.

    C. any of various procedures performed during cardiac catheterization, such as angioscopy and atherectomy.

    D. membranous muscle between the abdominal and thoracic cavities that contracts and relaxes during the respiratory cycle.

Circle the letter of the Question Combining Forms that corresponds to the displayed Answer.

11. glucose

    A. phantom limbs; phantom pain

    B. gluc(o)

    C. pansinusitis

    D. ischi(o)

12. bones that help form the hard palate and nasal cavity; located behind the maxillary bones.

    A. trich(o)

    B. peripheral vascular disease

    C. palatine bone

    D. epididymitis

13. conjunctiva

    A. miotic

    B. cystectomy

    C. conjunctiv(o)

    D. bi-

14. Inflammation of the esophagus
    A. resectoscope
    B. optician
    C. esophagitis
    D. scotoma

15. thorax
    A. petechia(pl. petechiae)
    B. cystoscope
    C. phosphorus
    D. thorac(o)

16. Removal of dead tissue from a wound.
    A. anthracosis
    B. ischium
    C. debridement
    D. peripheral vascular disease

17. bone with an open latticework filled with connective tissue or marrow.
    A. spongy bone
    B. apnea
    C. plastic surgery
    D. copulation

18. otitis media
    A. append(o), appendic(o)
    B. gastritis
    C. tox(o), toxi, toxico
    D. OM

19. Breaking of kidney stones by using shock waves from outside the body
    A. extracorporeal shock wave lithotripsy (ESWL)
    B. endothelium
    C. TPN
    D. anus

20. Disease caused by failure of the body to recognize insulin that is present or by abnormally low leve of insulin; also known as noninsulin-dependent diabetes mellitus (NIDDM); usually adult onset
    A. pineal gland
    B. hysteroctomy
    C. diabetes mellitus
    D. radiation therapy

EXTRA CREDIT: Give the Question Combining Forms that corresponds to the displayed Answer.

21. Urinary incontinence

Medical Definitions Quiz

Circle the letter of the Answer that corresponds to the displayed Question Combining Forms.

1. -plasm
    - A. formation
    - B. lip
    - C. insulin-dependent diabetes mellitus
    - D. egg

2. eyelashes
    - A. Group of hairs protruding from the end of the eyelid; helps to keep foreign particles from entering the eye
    - B. various substances located in tiny sacs at the end of the axon
    - C. X-ray image made after indroduction of a contrast medium and while urination is taking place
    - D. cancer

3. perineum
    - A. same; constant
    - B. Area between the penis and the anus
    - C. without tone; relaxed
    - D. Snail-shaped structure in the inner ear that contains the organ of Corti

4. pancreas
    - A. cell
    - B. magnetic resonance angiography
    - C. plasma
    - D. Digestive organ that secretes digestive fluids; endocrine gland that regulates blood sugar

5. blood
    - A. Disease caused by failure of the body to recognize insulin that is present or by abnormally low leve of insulin; also known as noninsulin-dependent diabetes mellitus (NIDDM); usually adult onset
    - B. Removal of the prostate
    - C. Three-to-five-year period of decreasing estrogen levels prior to menopause
    - D. Fluid (containing plasma, red blood cells, white blood cells, and platelets) circulated throughout the arteries, veins, capillaries, and heart

6. keratolytic
    - A. X-ray of the urethra and prostate
    - B. age-related macular degeneration
    - C. Agent that aids in the removal of warts and corns.
    - D. sugars

7. septostomy

A. Incision of the nasal septum
B. surgical replacement of a coronary valve.
C. fleshy tissue; muscle
D. arteriosclerotic cardiovascular disease

8. immun(o)
   A. dry
   B. turning toward
   C. immunity
   D. opening

9. spin(o)
   A. Group of ducts at the top of the testis where sperm are stored
   B. lateral, to one side
   C. movement
   D. spine

10. spermatozoon (pl. spermatozoa)
    A. Male sex cell that contains chromosomes
    B. hardening into bone.
    C. One of the parts of the diencephalon; serves as a sensory relay station
    D. Time when menstruation ceases; usually between ages 45 and 55

Circle the letter of the Question Combining Forms that corresponds to the displayed Answer.

11. Sense of balance
    A. pelvic cavity
    B. osteaglia
    C. cardiac MRI
    D. equilibrium

12. external, on the outside
    A. exo-
    B. AH
    C. -trophy
    D. gangliitis

13. Excessive urination
    A. osteoblast
    B. ca
    C. polyuria
    D. multiple sclerosis (MS)

14. Painful sexaul intercourse due to any of various conditions, such as cysts, infection, or dryness, in the vagina
    A. dyspareunia
    B. short bones
    C. -plasty
    D. ischi(o)

15. abnormal narrowing at the opening of the mitral valve.
    A. SPECT (single photon emission computed tomography) brain scan
    B. LLL
    C. mitral stenosis
    D. diphtheria

16. lack if flow through a blood vessel, usually caused by an occlusion.
    A. arthography
    B. perfusion deficit
    C. trachea(o)
    D. nephro(o)

17. minus/concave
    A. -
    B. ethmo
    C. tibia
    D. bucc(o)

18. Bottom lobe of the lung
    A. inferior lobe
    B. systemic lupus erythematosus
    C. AIDS
    D. spermatozoon (pl. spermatozoa)

19. artery
    A. medulla oblongata
    B. joint
    C. arteri(o) arter(o)
    D. LDH

20. Darkish area surrounding the nipple on a breast
    A. dextr(o)
    B. exocrine gland
    C. gastroenteritis
    D. areola

EXTRA CREDIT: Give the Question Combining Forms that corresponds to the displayed Answer.

21. wasting away

Medical Definitions Quiz

Circle the letter of the Answer that corresponds to the displayed Question Combining Forms.

1. mineralocorticoid
    - A. Steroid secreted by adrenal cortex
    - B. immunoglobulin A
    - C. Agent that removes excess oils and impurities from the surface of skin.
    - D. activated partial thromboplastin time

2. percussion
    - A. Injection of donor blood into a person needing blood
    - B. Tapping on the surface of the body to see if lungs are clear
    - C. long middle section of a long bone; shaft
    - D. Popping sounds heard in lung collapse or other conditions; rales

3. electrodesiccation
    - A. lymph nodes
    - B. rod-shaped
    - C. Drying with electrical current.
    - D. Loss of consciousness due to a sudden lack of oxygen to the brain

4. bone marrow biopsy
    - A. Mechanical breathing device
    - B. attacks of limping, particularly in the legs, due to ischemia of the muscles.
    - C. spine
    - D. Extraction of bone marrow, by means of a needle for observation

5. agnosia
    - A. Inability to receive and understand outside stimuli
    - B. plaque
    - C. curved
    - D. thin layer of keratin that covers the distal portion of fingers and toes.

6. talipes varus
    - A. joint of the lower jaw between the temporal bone and the mandible.
    - B. cessation of breathing
    - C. foot deformity characterized by inversion of the foot.
    - D. Removal of a testicle

7. polypectomy

    A. half
    B. tumor, neoplasm
    C. Removal of polyps
    D. Substance in the brain or manufactured substance that helps relieve symptoms of Parkinson's disease

8. bursitis
    A. inflammation of bursa
    B. Darkish area surrounding the nipple on a breast
    C. Inflammation of the kidneys
    D. Agent that lowers blood glucose

9. pyelitis
    A. sheet of fibrous tissue connecting and supporting bones; attaches bone to bone.
    B. follicle-stimulating hormone
    C. Inflammation of the renal pelvis
    D. Cartilaginous division, as in the nose or mediastinum

10. angiotensin converting enzyme inhibitor
    A. Eye with an implanted lens after cataract surgery
    B. Malignant kidney tumor found primarily in young children; nephroblastoma
    C. chronic lymphocytic leukemia
    D. medication used for heart failure and other cardiovascular problems; acts by dilating arteries to lower blood pressure and makes heart pump easier.

Circle the letter of the Question Combining Forms that corresponds to the displayed Answer.

11. Agent that relieves the symptoms of inflammations.
    A. -gram
    B. lymphadenectomy
    C. acetabul(o)
    D. anti-inflammatory

12. Hereditary disease that causes deterioration in the central nervous system and eventually, death
    A. constriction
    B. inferior
    C. Tay-Sachs disease
    D. perineum

13. tissue
    A. angioplasty
    B. hyperbilirubinemia
    C. anticonvulsant
    D. histi(o), histo

14. Large masses of gray matter within the cerebrum
    A. angioplasty
    B. basal ganglia
    C. cystic fibrosis
    D. otitis media

15. Pigment contained in bile
    A. bilirubin
    B. menorrhagia
    C. uric acid test
    D. orthopedist

16. body system that forms and excretes urine and helps in the reabsorption of essential substances
    A. urinary system
    B. voice box
    C. sub-
    D. fluor(o)

17. Establsihment of an opening from the renal pelvis to the outside of the body
    A. diopter
    B. acquired immunodeficiency disease
    C. nephrostomy
    D. gallstones

18. Incompatibility disoreder between a mother with Rh negative and a fetus with Rh positive
    A. urethrotomy
    B. blindness
    C. ABG
    D. erythroblastosis fetalis

19. enlargement
    A. bronchial alveolar lavage
    B. orchiectomy
    C. -megaly
    D. nas(O)

20. Body space that contains the spinal cord.
    A. cec(o)
    B. spinal cavity
    C. metaphysis
    D. -para

EXTRA CREDIT: Give the Question Combining Forms that corresponds to the displayed Answer.
21. Backward flow from the normal direction

Medical Definitions Quiz

Circle the letter of the Answer that corresponds to the displayed Question Combining Forms.

1. hilum
    - A. Agent that relieves feeling of agitation
    - B. Disposable catheter for urinary sample collection or incontinence
    - C. Portion of the kidney where blood vessels and nerves enter and exit
    - D. abdomen

2. spermicide
    - A. Incision into the trachea
    - B. left ventricular hypertrophy
    - C. Nighttime urination
    - D. Contraceptive chemical that destroys sperm; usually in cream or jelly form

3. plasma, plasmo, plasmat(o)
    - A. valve that controls the blood flow between the right ventricle and the pulmonary arteries.
    - B. plasma
    - C. nosogastric
    - D. Yellowish-brown to greenish fluid secreted by the liver and stored in the gallbladder; aids in fat digestion

4. casts
    - A. Jaundice
    - B. materials formed in urine when protein accumlates; may indicate renal disease
    - C. right lower lobe (of the lungs)
    - D. Chemical secretion from glands such as the ovaries

5. inferior vena cava
    - A. large vein that draws blood from the lower part of the body to the right atrium.
    - B. lower left heart chamber
    - C. Medical doctor who diagnoses and treats disorders of the ear, nose and throat
    - D. cecum

6. Inhibiting
    - A. Protein that aids in forming a fibrin clot
    - B. Preventin the secretion of other hormones
    - C. Part of a nerve cell that has branches or fibers that reach out to send or receive impulses
    - D. cystoscopy

7. bilirubin

A. Pigment contained in bile
B. polymorphonuclear neurtrophil
C. Organ of lymph system that filters, stores, removes, blood, and activates lymphocytes
D. right, toward the right

8. -phoria
    A. iris
    B. feeling; carrying
    C. Agent that lowers blood glucose
    D. Mature white blood cell

9. halitosis
    A. heel bone
    B. Foul mouth odor
    C. one of twenty-four bones that form the chest wall.
    D. Examination of the colon using an endoscope

10. mammary glands
    A. muscles not movable at will.
    B. Passageway at back of mouth for air and food; throat
    C. Birth defect with abnormal opening of the urethra on the top side of the penis
    D. Glandular tissue that forms the breasts, which respond to cycles of menstuation and birth

Circle the letter of the Question Combining Forms that corresponds to the displayed Answer.

11. Gland in the nervous system that releases hormones to aid in regulating pituitary hormones
    A. rhinitis
    B. osteoma
    C. filtration
    D. hypothalamus

12. without, outside of
    A. extra-
    B. arthroscopy
    C. gallbladder
    D. autograft

13. spine
    A. macule
    B. epispadias
    C. spin(o)
    D. cortisol

14. Body system that includes muscles, bones, and cartilage.
    A. gonio
    B. urethrogram
    C. musculoskeletal system
    D. aerotitis media

15. maxilla
    A. maxill(o)
    B. normo
    C. external nares
    D. GOT

16. cause
    A. TAH-BSO
    B. etio
    C. ENT
    D. chancroids

17. Removal or destruction of tissue using cold temperatures
    A. STH
    B. Babinski's reflex
    C. xenograft
    D. cryosurgery

18. Endocrine gland
    A. otoscopy
    B. ductless gland
    C. PMS
    D. mammoplasty

19. small bone consisting of four fused vertebrae at the end of the spinal column; tailbone
    A. exotropia
    B. coccyx
    C. spinal nerves
    D. -emic

20. right upper lobe (of the lungs)
    A. gonio
    B. ur(o) urin(o)
    C. RUL
    D. pyelotomy

EXTRA CREDIT: Give the Question Combining Forms that corresponds to the displayed Answer.
21. thick scarring of the skin that forms after an injury or surgery.

Medical Definitions Quiz

Circle the letter of the Answer that corresponds to the displayed Question Combining Forms.

1. spir(o)
    - A. Hormone given to stop labor
    - B. breath; breathe
    - C. Outer portion of the skin containing several strata
    - D. tarsus

2. epidural space
    - A. Reversal of a vasectomy
    - B. Area between the pia mater and the bones of the spinal cord
    - C. disease that causes a viral skin rash; measles.
    - D. Removal of dead tissue from a wound.

3. diff
    - A. retina
    - B. death of portions of bone.
    - C. differential blood count
    - D. Simple protein; when leaked into urine, may indicate a kidney problem

4. lactation
    - A. slow
    - B. Production of milk from the breasts following delivery
    - C. Condition caused by the abnormal release of ketones in the body
    - D. fluid that serves to lubricate joints.

5. heart
    - A. air sac, alveolus
    - B. musclar organ that receives blood from the veins and sends it into the arteries.
    - C. Suturing of a severed nerve
    - D. Left and right regions of the body near the upper portion of the hip bone.

6. A&P
    - A. chronic lymphocytic leukemia
    - B. auscultation and percussion
    - C. cheek
    - D. bundles of fibers in the interventricular septum that transfer charges in the heart's conduction system; also called bundle of His.

7. osteoplasty

A. surgical replacement or repair of bone.
   B. immunoglobulin G
   C. viewing of the heart and its major blood vessel by x-ray after injection of a contrast medium.
   D. Specialized protein that fights disease

8. radioactive iodine therapy
   A. Type of virus that spreads by using DNA in the body to help it replicate its RNA
   B. Use of radioactive iodine to eliminate thyroid tumors
   C. Pouch at the top of the large intestine connected to the bottom of the ileum
   D. both ears

9. ophthalm(o
   A. eye
   B. Removal of the testicles
   C. metacarpal
   D. derived. separate

10. Papanicolaou smear
    A. Gathering of cells from the cervix and vagina to abserve for abnormalities
    B. Medication to prevent implantation of an ovum
    C. Deviation of one eye inward
    D. wrist

Circle the letter of the Question Combining Forms that corresponds to the displayed Answer.

11. abnormal lateral curvature of the spinal column.
    A. gait
    B. aer(o)
    C. scoliosis
    D. IBS

12. chronic condition with obstruction or narrowing of the bronchial airways.
    A. semilunar valve
    B. thymectomy
    C. asthma
    D. contra-

13. pain in the lower back, usually radiating down the leg, from a herniated disk or other injury or condition.
    A. interneuron
    B. exanthematous viral disease
    C. pyreto
    D. sciatica

14. ultrasound test of blood flow in certain vessels.
    A. PEEP
    B. doppler ultrasound
    C. myelogram
    D. OM

15. Sexual intercourse
    A. inferior lobe
    B. tinnitus
    C. coitus
    D. angiography

16. against
    A. contra-
    B. oligodendroglia
    C. laryng(o)
    D. maxill(o)

17. viscera
    A. pulmonary vein
    B. mastoid(o)
    C. splanchn(o), splanchni
    D. pancreat(o)

18. glucose
    A. Bright's disease
    B. -genesis
    C. ascites
    D. gluc(o)

19. Specialized cells that produce insulin in the pancreas
    A. beta cells
    B. retroflexion
    C. thrombocytopenia
    D. hemi-

20. injury to a muscle as a result of overuse.
    A. blood
    B. myasthenia gravis
    C. strain
    D. gastroenteritis

EXTRA CREDIT: Give the Question Combining Forms that corresponds to the displayed Answer.
21. Condition with an abnormal number of eosinophils in the blood

Medical Definitions Test

Enter the letter for the matching Answer

1. ☐ gastrectomy
2. ☐ -stomy
3. ☐ melanin
4. ☐ blood system
5. ☐ menarche
6. ☐ acetabul(o)
7. ☐ LDH
8. ☐ puberty
9. ☐ nocturia
10. ☐ ovi, ovo
11. ☐ azoospermia
12. ☐ chem(o)
13. ☐ distal
14. ☐ end-stage-renal disease (ESRD)
15. ☐ osteopath
16. ☐ ca
17. ☐ miscarriage
18. ☐ tox(o), toxi, toxico
19. ☐ EMG
20. ☐ connective tissue

A. Spontaneous, premature ending of a pregnancy
B. lactate dehydroganase
C. chemical
D. opening
E. electromyogram
F. acetabulum
G. calcium
H. Body system that includes blood and all its component parts
I. egg; ova
J. Removal of part or all of the stomach
K. poison
L. Away from the point of attachment of the trunk.
M. The last stage of kidney failure
N. physician who combines manipulative treatment with conventional therapeutic measures.
O. Nighttime urination
P. pigment produced by melanocytes that determines skin, hair, and eye color.
Q. Semen without living sperm
R. Pre-teen or early teen period when secondary sex characteristics develop and menstruation begins
S. Fibrous substance that forms the body's supportive framework.
T. First menstruation

Give the Answer that corresponds to the displayed Question Combining Forms.

21. erythr(o)

22. dia-

23. dys-

Give the Question Combining Forms that corresponds to the displayed Answer.

24. large cells that reabsorbs and removes osseous tissue.

25. condition that reduces the flow of blood and nutrients through the arteries of the heart.

26. Visual examination of the interior of the eye

27. One of two male organs that secretes hormones in the endocrine system

28. an irregular, usually rapid, heartbeat caused by overstimulation of the AV node.

29. Process of returning essential elements to the bloodstream after filtration

30. coiled glands of the skin that secrete perspiration to regulate body temperature and excrete waste products.

Medical Definitions Test

Enter the letter for the matching Answer

1. ☐ -philia
2. ☐ IM
3. ☐ vomer
4. ☐ empyema
5. ☐ trich(o)
6. ☐ col(o), colon(o)
7. ☐ calcane(o)
8. ☐ scler(o)
9. ☐ -static
10. ☐ pelvis
11. ☐ trachel(o)
12. ☐ bursitis
13. ☐ dislocation
14. ☐ patch
15. ☐ Ach
16. ☐ ecchymosis (pl. ecchymoses)
17. ☐ phon(o)
18. ☐ ICCE
19. ☐ esophag(o)
20. ☐ PSA

A. esophagus
B. intramuscularly
C. movement of a joint out of its normal position as a result of an injury or sudden, strenuous movement.
D. attraction; affinity for
E. cup-shaped ring of bone and ligaments at the base of the trunk.
F. intracapsular cataract cryoextraction
G. flat bone forming the nasal septum
H. pus in the pleural cavity
I. acetylcholine
J. inflammation of bursa
K. maintaining a state
L. heel bone
M. small area of skin differing in color from the surrounding area.
N. prostate-specific antigen
O. white of the eye
P. Purplish skin patch(bruise) caused by broken blood vessels beneath the surface.
Q. sound; voice; speech
R. hair
S. neck
T. colon

Give the Answer that corresponds to the displayed Question Combining Forms.

21. meg(a), megal(o)

22. ovari(o)

Give the Question Combining Forms that corresponds to the displayed Answer.

23. Tissue that covers or lines the body or its parts.

24. muscle pain

25. coiled glands of the skin that secrete perspiration to regulate body temperature and excrete waste products.

26. Bleeding condition with insufficient production of platelets

27. Elvated pressure within the cochlea

28. Measure of the intensity of sound

29. See urticaria group of reddish wheals, usually accompanied by pruritus and often caused by an allergy.

30. foot deformity characterized by inversion of the foot.

Medical Definitions Test

Enter the letter for the matching Answer

1. ☐ orchidectomy
2. ☐ nephritis
3. ☐ suppressor cell
4. ☐ atheroma
5. ☐ hepat(o)
6. ☐ striated muscle
7. ☐ glossectomy
8. ☐ test(o)
9. ☐ anabolic steriods
10. ☐ scoli(o)
11. ☐ coni(o)
12. ☐ cervic(o)
13. ☐ pyel(o)
14. ☐ greenstick fracture
15. ☐ Type II diabetes
16. ☐ semilunar valve
17. ☐ hirsutism
18. ☐ connective tissue
19. ☐ SA
20. ☐ eupnea

A. Inflammation of the kidneys
B. muscle with a ribbed appearance that is controlled at will.
C. a fatty deposit (plaque) in the wall of an artery.
D. Removal of the tongue
E. liver
F. one of the two valves that prevent the backflow of blood flowing out of the heart into the aorta and the pulmonary artery.
G. Abnormal hair growth due to an excess of androgens
H. Fibrous substance that forms the body's supportive framework.
I. Prescription drug abused by some athletes to increase muscle mass
J. Removal of a testicle
K. dust
L. neck;cervix
M. renal pelvis
N. curved
O. normal breathing
P. fracture with twisting or bending of the bone but no breaking; usually occurs in children.
Q. sinoatrial
R. testis
S. Disease caused by failure of the body to recognize insulin that is present or by abnormally low leve of insulin; also known as noninsulin-dependent diabetes mellitus (NIDDM); usually adult onset
T. t cell that suppresses B cells and other immune cells

Give the Answer that corresponds to the displayed Question Combining Forms.

21. visceral muscle

22. odont(o)

23. ren(o)

24. pyreto

Give the Question Combining Forms that corresponds to the displayed Answer.

25. drugs; medicine

26. Specialized receptors cells withing the taste buds

27. Inability to swallow

28. pain

29. Removal of the frontal lobe of the brain

30. Absence of lens

Medical Definitions Test

Enter the letter for the matching Answer

1. ☐ neuroplasty
2. ☐ kinesi(o), kineso
3. ☐ SOM
4. ☐ ethmoid sinuses
5. ☐ Bell's palsy
6. ☐ right lower quadrant (RLQ)
7. ☐ DJD
8. ☐ hematocrit
9. ☐ sciatica
10. ☐ gravida
11. ☐ immun(o)
12. ☐ PND
13. ☐ cell body
14. ☐ VA
15. ☐ septum
16. ☐ digestion
17. ☐ keratolytic
18. ☐ gluc(o)
19. ☐ laryng(o)
20. ☐ VT

A. Conversion of food into nutrients for the body and into waste products for release from the body

B. Part of a nerve cell that has branches or fibers that reach out to send or receive impulses

C. Pregnant woman

D. ventricular tachycardia

E. pain in the lower back, usually radiating down the leg, from a herniated disk or other injury or condition.

F. Surgical repair of a nerve

G. serious otitis media

H. degenerative joint disease

I. sinuses on both sides of the nasal cavities between each eye and the sphenoid sinus.

J. glucose

K. partition between the left and right chambers of the heart

L. visual acuity

M. Measure of the percentage of red blood cells in a blood sample

N. Agent that aids in the removal of warts and corns.

O. immunity

P. larynx

Q. paroxysmal nocturnal dyspnea; postnasal drip

R. Paralysis of one side of the face; usually temporary

S. motion

T. Quadrant on the lower right anterior side of the patient's body

Give the Answer that corresponds to the displayed Question Combining Forms.

21. gangli(o)

Give the Question Combining Forms that corresponds to the displayed Answer.

22. Inflammation of the small intestine

23. grapelike clusters

24. inflammation of the epiglottis

25. endotracheal intubation tube

26. procedure that uses a balloon catheter to open narrowed orifices in cardiac valves.

27. Surgical union of two hollow structures

28. depression, as in a bone.

29. fracture with twisting or bending of the bone but no breaking; usually occurs in children.

30. cystoscopy

Medical Definitions Test

Enter the letter for the matching Answer

1. ☐ un-
2. ☐ medulla oblongata
3. ☐ NG
4. ☐ atrial fibrillation
5. ☐ salpingectomy
6. ☐ glomerul(o)
7. ☐ transfusion
8. ☐ episi(o)
9. ☐ nonsteriodal anti-inflammatory drug
10. ☐ metr(o)
11. ☐ gyn(o), gyne, gyneco
12. ☐ HCG
13. ☐ heparin
14. ☐ lingu(o)
15. ☐ phag(o)
16. ☐ sty, stye
17. ☐ bypass
18. ☐ pancytopenia
19. ☐ sphygm(o)
20. ☐ epistaxis

A. an irregular, usually rapid, heartbeat caused by overstimulation of the AV node.

B. agent that reduces inflammation without the use of steroids.

C. eating, devouring

D. Condition with low number of blood components

E. glomerulus

F. not

G. Part of the brain stem that regulates hear and lung functions, swallowing, vomiting, coughing, and sneezing

H. bleeding from the nose, usually caused by trauma or a sudden rupture of the blood vessels of the nose.

I. a structure (usually a vein graft) that creates a new passage for blood to flow from one artery to another artery or part of an artery; used to create a detour around blockages in arteries.

J. tongue

K. uterus

L. human chorionic gonadotropin

M. anticoagulant present in the body; also, synthetic version administered to prevent clotting.

N. Injection of donor blood into a person needing blood

O. nosogastric

P. Hordeolum

Q. women

R. pulse

S. Removal of a fallopian tube

T. vulva

Give the Answer that corresponds to the displayed Question Combining Forms.

21. steth(o)

22. hypopharynx

23. mio

Give the Question Combining Forms that corresponds to the displayed Answer.

24. test for tuberculosis in which a small dose of tuberculin in injected into the skin with a syringe.

25. Abnormally low movement of air in out of the lungs.

26. Loss or absences of vision

27. light; luminous; fluorine

28. Abnormal reaction to an allergen

29. External openings or entrance to a hollow organ, such as a vagina

30. Abnormal growth of eyelashes in a direction that causes them rub on the eye

Printed in Great Britain
by Amazon